*Beverly A. Ogilvie, MA, RCC*

# Mother-Daughter Incest
## *A Guide*
## *for Helping Professionals*

*Pre-publication*
*REVIEWS,*
*COMMENTARIES,*
*EVALUATIONS . . .*

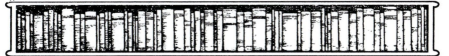

*More pre-publication*
*REVIEWS, COMMENTARIES, EVALUATIONS . . .*

"**O**gilvie gives voice to the previously voiceless victims of mother-daughter incest by sharing the stories and experiences of survivors. She shows how society has perpetuated the cover-up of this victimization through the idealization of motherhood and the mother-daughter relationship, as well as through the taboos imposed on both incest and homosexuality. With compassion and understanding, she opens the reader's eyes to the experiences of victims and the impact this rarely disclosed form of abuse has had on their lives.

With insight and sensitivity, the author provides a framework for therapists working with the victims of mother-daughter incest to help survivors move from a place of isolation, anguish, and shame to a place of strength, purpose, and pride."

**Sarah Robertson, RN**
*Child and Family Therapist,*
*Ministry of Children and Family*
*Development, North Burnaby,*
*British Columbia, Canada*

"**T**his book addresses the historical and cultural components that exacerbate the secrecy and denial of victims of mother-daughter incest. Ogilvie takes the reader deep into the multilayered impacts, and presents the intense, pervasive damage this abuse has on children. The book offers professional observations along with the voices of victims telling their personal stories, and even gives some space to the mother's experience. Ogilvie offers various counseling interventions, clearly and without judgment, by focusing on multifaceted aspects of designing a healing process tailored to each individual and her unique combination of trauma experiences."

**Naomi A. Serrano, PhD**
*Relationship and Family Therapist,*
*British Columbia, Canada*

**HMTP**

The Haworth Maltreatment and Trauma Press®
An Imprint of The Haworth Press, Inc.
New York • London • Oxford

# Mother-Daughter Incest
## *A Guide*
## *for Helping Professionals*

# Mother-Daughter Incest
## *A Guide*
## *for Helping Professionals*

Beverly A. Ogilvie, MA, RCC

**HMTP**

The Haworth Maltreatment and Trauma Press®
An Imprint of The Haworth Press, Inc.
New York • London • Oxford

Published by

The Haworth Maltreatment and Trauma Press®, an imprint of The Haworth Press, Inc., 10 Alice Street, Binghamton, NY 13904-1580.

PUBLISHER'S NOTE
Identities and circumstances of individuals discussed in this book have been changed to protect confidentiality.

Cover design by Lora Wiggins.

**Library of Congress Cataloging-in-Publication Data**

Ogilvie, Beverly A.
    Mother-daughter incest : a guide for helping professionals / Beverly A. Ogilvie.
        p. cm.
    Includes bibliographical references and index.
    ISBN 0-7890-0916-1 (case : alk. paper)—ISBN 0-7890-0917-X (soft : alk. paper)
    1. Incest. 2. Incest victims. 3. Abusive mothers. 4. Mothers and daughters. 5. Incest victims—Rehabilitation. 6. Adult child sexual abuse victims—Rehabilitation. I. Title.
HV6570.6.045 2004
362.76—dc22
                                                                                                    2003016143

For my father
Fleming Harry Ogilvie
(1921-2002)

With gratitude to

those mother-daughter incest survivors
who took the time to tell me their stories
and express their desire to assist others;
those mother-daughter incest survivors
who are silently enduring—
may you hear your own cry
in the cries of those who have told their stories
and receive their assistance;
the new, silent child victims—
may you break through your walls of secrecy and shame;
those who live, love, or work with mother-daughter
incest survivors—may you support their movement
from survivor to creator, from wounded to healed,
from part to whole, from disintegration to integration,
and from disconnected to connected.

## ABOUT THE AUTHOR

**Beverly A. Ogilvie, MA, RCC,** is District Special Secondary Counselor for School District #41 in Burnaby, British Columbia. She has twenty years of professional teaching experience in public schools as well as colleges and universities. She is a registered clinical counselor and a member of the British Columbia School Counselors Association. As an author and researcher, she has published materials and articles on the subject of mother-daughter incestuous abuse. Her most recent publication, "Why Didn't She Love Me? Mother-Daughter Incest: An Overview of the Effect on the Survivors," (1996) was a project completed for Health Canada's Family Violence Prevention Division.

# CONTENTS

Preface                                                           ix

Acknowledgments                                                   xi

## PART I: THE ENIGMA OF MOTHER-DAUGHTER INCEST                   1

Chapter 1. Introduction                                           3

Chapter 2. The Essential Human Connection                       11

## PART II: COMMON THEMES AMONG DAUGHTERS                        25

Chapter 3. Acute Shame                                          27

Chapter 4. Trapped with No Place to Go                          37

Chapter 5. Double-Crossed: Betrayal and Grief                  45

Chapter 6. Identification with and Differentiation from Mother  55

Chapter 7. Impaired Sexual Development                          63

Chapter 8. Difficulty Coping                                    71

## PART III: COMMON THEMES AMONG MOTHERS                         83

Chapter 9. Emotionally Needy and Unstable Mothers              85

Chapter 10. Boundary Violations                                93

## PART IV: SPECIFIC COUNSELING INTERVENTIONS                   101

Chapter 11. Stigmatization                                     103

Chapter 12. Identity Development                               109

Chapter 13. Parenting                                          119

Chapter 14. Treating the Adult Victim                         123

PART V: SPECIAL ISSUES                                        133

Chapter 15. Stepmothers versus Biological Mothers            135

Chapter 16. Therapist Gender                                 139

Chapter 17. Transference                                     145

Chapter 18. Countertransference                              155

Chapter 19. Theoretical Frameworks and Treatment
    Approaches                           171

Chapter 20. Conclusion                                       181

Bibliography                                                 185

Index                                                        193

# Preface

The majority of the sexual abuse literature has focused on male-perpetrated abuse or primarily father-daughter incest. Until recently, mother-child incest was considered to be virtually nonexistent.

As a society, we have become quite compartmentalized in terms of thinking concerning who is a victim and who is an abuser. Our current view of who abuses and who is victimized has its roots in the women's movement and continues to be shaped by a consciousness that tells only part of the abuse/survivor story. As a result, the experiences of other persons outside this model have been overlooked. Their voices have been muted. Their silence remains!

Very few resources are presently available for mother-daughter incest survivors that, by the nature of the topic, serve to challenge this mode or historically shaped consciousness. Survivors of mother-daughter incest have had their experiences kept outside of public and professional discourse on sexual abuse. Their voices have yet to be added to the consciousness. As such, *Mother-Daughter Incest: A Guide for Helping Professionals* makes an important contribution to the literature and therapeutic practice; the voices of women who have been sexually abused at the hands of their mothers will be added to the dialogue on sexual abuse in a significant way.

*Mother-Daughter Incest: A Guide for Helping Professionals* was written to fill this gap in the literature. The intention of the book is to expand consciousness and change beliefs about sexual abuse by exploring the phenomenon of mother-daughter incest. Sexual abuse by mothers needs to be acknowledged as a reality in the lives of some women.

This book provides descriptions of the phenomenon of mother-daughter incest and expands knowledge about the differing dynamics entailed in the incest relationship based on the gender of the abuser. It does not pay a great deal of attention to the mothers' motivations for perpetrating the abuse but primarily emphasizes the victims' perceptions and reactions to their experiences of incest at the hands of their mothers. Similarities with other types of sexual abuse are addressed, as are problems specific to mother-daughter incest survivors.

The goal of this book is to sensitize researchers and practitioners to the nature and meaning of the experience of mother-daughter incest, help contradict prevalent misconceptions about incest, and decrease social and personal denial of such abuse. By providing accurate information about mother-daughter incest, its manifestations and unique dynamics, the clinician will be able to plan and focus treatment so that the special needs of mother-daughter incest survivors may be better met.

This book provides introductory information about factors that contribute to the underreporting and underinvestigation of the phenomenon of mother-daughter incest. The significance of the mother-daughter bond, in particular cultural definitions and expectations of motherhood, is explored as key factors in societal denial of the existence of mother-daughter incest.

Based on my research with over sixty adult female survivors of sexual abuse at the hands of their mothers and informed by the literature in the area (albeit scarce in nature), this book focuses on the experience of mother-daughter incest from the daughter's perspective. Emphasis is placed on common themes extracted from the research data, some of which parallel the experience of survivors of other forms of sexual abuse and some which are more specific to mother-daughter incest. Separate chapters are dedicated to the discussion of salient themes, supported by dialogue from the participants where possible. The women's own words are used to help articulate their experiences of sexual abuse at the hands of their mothers, their past and present relationships with their mothers, and their perceptions of the impact of the abuse on their lives. Names and identifying data have been altered to ensure anonymity. This book incorporates developmental and attachment theories along with trauma models to provide the context within which the manifestations and unique dynamics of mother-daughter incest are better understood. Implications for therapeutic practice are explored throughout the book, and treatment recommendations are made for helping professionals working with incest survivors of maternal sexual abuse.

# Acknowledgments

To my best friend, Karen Meier, who lovingly and enthusiastically supported me throughout the writing of this book. I am especially grateful for her invaluable assistance in typing and retyping the manuscript.

To my parents, Fleming and Evelyn Ogilvie, for their confidence in me, and their undying love and emotional support during the various stages of preparing this book.

To my friends and professional colleagues, notably Laurie McGillivray, Joanna Doonan, Barrie Pollock, and Sarah Robertson, for their encouragement and insight throughout this project. Special thanks to Don Macdonald, Terry Waterhouse, Deb Simak, and other Burnaby School District staff for their ongoing support.

To my twin sister, Brenda Flanders, who has always been there for me and has always been totally supportive of all my endeavors. I thank her for her love and friendship.

To my nephew, Brodie Flanders, to whom I've been a surrogate mom these past two years. He is my inspiration. He has modeled for me what it is to follow one's dreams and enjoy the ride.

To Adam Tulk, to whom I've also been a guardian these past two years. I am inspired by his drive and determination to be the best and to accomplish his goals.

I am indebted to Bob Geffner, my editor, for his suggestions, knowledge, and guidance during the writing of this book.

# PART I:
# THE ENIGMA
# OF MOTHER-DAUGHTER INCEST

The significance of the mother-daughter relationship, in particular cultural images of motherhood, contributes to societal denial that mothers may sexually abuse their daughters, and to the underestimation and underreporting of the phenomenon of mother-daughter incest. Developmental and attachment theories provide a context in which the impact of mother-daughter incest may be better understood.

# Chapter 1

# Introduction

Females are more likely than males to be victims of childhood sexual abuse. Finkelhor and Browne (1985) estimate that roughly 70 percent of sexual abuse victims are female. Sexual abuse of females starts earlier than does abuse of males, and females are more likely than males to be assaulted by a family member. As a consequence, their abuse lasts longer, causes more severe trauma, and causes dramatic short- and long-term effects (Russell, 1984; Finkelhor and Browne, 1985; Chesney-Lind, 1997).

According to the Bureau of Justice Statistics (1997), the number of sexual assault crimes more than doubled from 1990 to 1996. Men accounted for 98 percent of the total arrested for these sexual assaults. Sex offenses by females (except forcible rape and prostitution) increased by a rate of 10.9 percent between 1985 and 1994 (Bureau of Justice Statistics, 1997), and those females arrested were usually accomplices to the crime. Female sex offenders have been described in the literature (Maison and Larson, 1995) as being victims of extreme childhood abuse, having unmet emotional needs, and being completely dependent on men who initiate abuse. They lack compulsive sexual fantasies about children (compared to male sex offenders) and are strangely unconcerned about the loss of parental rights. They often choose to seduce children, and they plan unrealistic futures with their child lovers (van Wormer, 2001).

Despite the increase in research into what was once a taboo subject, information still tends to be limited to specific areas of child sexual abuse, notably interfamilial sexual abuse and sexual abuse of females by male perpetrators (opposite-sex abuse). Society remains ignorant about the lives of female offenders. Estimates of female-perpetrated child sexual abuse based on a variety of surveys of the general population (Blanchard, 1987; Finkelhor et al., 1989; O'Hagan, 1989; Russell, 1984) place the percentage of sexual contacts by females at 20 percent (14 to 27 percent range) for male children and approximately 5 percent (0 to 10 percent range) for female children. Little information exists on the prevalence and consequences of same-sex (male-male or female-female) abuse.

Although the research evidence still indicates that fathers are most frequently the perpetrators of incestuous abuse and daughters are most frequently their victims (Browne and Finkelhor, 1986; Courtois, 1988), some mothers also cross the boundaries of sexual abuse with their children (Banning, 1989; Johnson and Shrier, 1987; Ogilvie and Daniluk, 1995; Ogilvie, 1996; Rosencrans, 1997). New research and clinical evidence indicates that mothers, in larger numbers than had previously been indicated, may be accomplices to or co-offenders in father-child incest or may be sole perpetrators with children of either sex.

Recent research suggests that mother-daughter incest is not rare; it is underestimated and underreported because its occurrence involves the breaking of two taboos, incest and homosexuality. In a homophobic society such as ours, a mother's incestuous wishes toward daughters are far more forbidden and shameful than toward sons. Mother-daughter incest is a greater moral taboo than other types of family incest. Because confusion exists in the literature regarding prevalence rates of child abuse, and also because little is known about mother-daughter incest, incidence data on mother-daughter incest are virtually nonexistent.

Several factors contribute to the underestimation and underreporting of the phenomenon and to the dearth of available information that addresses the dynamics and sequelae of mother-daughter incest, including

- societal denial of the possibility that mothers may sexually exploit their children;
- cultural images of motherhood; and
- stigmatization.

Particular attention needs to be given to the significance of the mother-daughter relationship in terms of current conceptions of mother as primary protector, gentle, passive, and nurturing, as well as predominant cultural images of motherhood as contributors to the controversy surrounding the incidence of sexual abuse by mothers.

## SOCIETAL DENIAL

Little attention has been given in the media and in professional arenas to the issue of sexual abuse of children by females. Female pedophilia has been reported in the literature as infrequent, and female sex offenders have rarely been studied and are poorly understood. Only within the past decade has society started to pay attention to the problem of sexual abuse and to the dynamics of male victims. Inadvertently, with this increased media and professional attention, increases in the estimated numbers of female sex offenders have been discovered. Still, the extent of sexual abuse by females remains a controversial issue. Society continues to assume that very few females are perpetrators due to general disbelief that this can occur. Many researchers contend that sexual abuse by females is far from an uncommon experience.

It appears that incest by a male/father is viewed by our society as more normal and acceptable than similar behaviors perpetrated by a female/mother. The feminist community has been especially reluctant to acknowledge factors other than patriarchy in the etiology of abuse. Because of gender and sexual scripts found in patriarchal families, girls are much more likely than boys to be victims of family-related sexual abuse. Men are more likely to consider their daughters or stepdaughters as their sexual property (van Wormer, 2001; Chesney-Lind, 1997). As a society, we are operating a double standard or an asymmetrical incest taboo. We take it for granted that men/fathers abuse, yet we refuse to accept that women/mothers sexually abuse as well. Public outrage against female perpetrators reflects society's contradictory expectations of women. It is not surprising, then, that society responds to sexual abuse by mothers with extreme discomfort, shock, and disbelief. We have reached the point where we can talk about rape, spousal abuse, and father-son incest, but we turn away from mother-daughter incest.

Gilbert and Webster (1982) address the "trap of daughterhood" which has definite implications for the notion of parental abuse of daughters. They define the family as a "sovereign nation" which expects, especially from its daughters, an oath of fidelity that predicates and idealizes everything that transpires within familial borders. The daughter is expected to join the parents in promoting the rules that maintain family unity. She is expected to identify with her mother because of inevitable role modeling, yet she fears familial exile and being thrust out of the emotional familiarity of the family. She has little choice but to take the oath and accept the consequences of hierarchy and inequality built into daily life. Daughters are expected to obey the adults who supposedly act in their interest. Parents, in particular mothers, are entrusted with the responsibility of nurturing and protecting their children from the dangers of their physically and socially powerless position. From this perspective, bound by love and duty, gratitude and fear, the daughter can only hope that her parents, in particular her mother, with whom she identifies the most, comprehend and respect the boundaries of childhood.

One might argue that the "trap of parenthood" also exists. Societal expectations assume parents, in particular mothers, will act with constraint, tempering their absolute power with mercy and love. Societal definitions of motherhood continue to view mothers as incapable of perpetrating sexual abuse and as somehow "morally better than men" (Rosencrans, 1997, p. 238). Society still perpetuates the myth that nice families, in white houses with picket fences, are problem-free and void of dysfunction. In no way has society been ready to accept that mothers are in any way capable of engineering a terrible disruption of attachment that maternal abuse creates.

## *CULTURAL IMAGES OF MOTHERHOOD*

Women, and in particular mothers, are not viewed as sexual, violent, or aggressive, but rather as gentle, passive, and nonsexual. Mothers are expected to nurture and rear children with warmth, caring, and guidance. To confront the knowledge that a mother, the primary protector, is abusive to her child, much less sexually abusive, is to profoundly challenge our cultural images of motherhood.

The mother-child relationship is the first and most fundamental relationship for the child. Society tolerates a greater degree of closeness, of physical intimacy, between mothers and daughters, thereby making recognition of incestuous acts more difficult. Socially accepted physical intimacy between a mother and her daughter may serve to mask inappropriate sexual acts on the part of the mother. These mothers are not acknowledged by society and therefore are free to abuse with almost total impunity. As victims of mother-daughter incest, and members of a society that has denied the existence of the phenomenon of mother-daughter incest, survivors of maternal abuse are unable to speak about the unspeakable.

An obvious relationship exists, then, between a cultural context which largely denies the possibility that a woman might sexually abuse a child, in particular her daughter, and the underreporting and underinvestigation of the phenomenon of mother-daughter incest. The taboo and enforced silence that has historically surrounded the phenomenon of mother-daughter incest sets the stage for a climate of secrecy. So huge is their secret that these women cannot share the dreaded truth for fear that, because it is so forbidden by society, it would drive away the few individuals they trust.

## *STIGMATIZATION*

Stigma is defined as a mark of shame or discredit, a trace, scar, blot, stain, mark, brand, or vestige. Mother-daughter incest survivors often report that the sexual abuse they experienced at the hands of their mothers is the most hidden aspect of their lives. During their childhood, the majority of mother-daughter incest victims do not tell anyone about their abuse. A survey of ninety-three survivors completed by Rosencrans (1997) addresses the extent of the silence experienced by mother-daughter incest survivors in that the average wait before telling anyone about their abuse was twenty-eight years.

Mother-daughter incest survivors describe their sexual abuse as shameful and stigmatizing due to the uniqueness of the experience and the isolation of the abuse. For many victims, a dearth of information about the issue and a lack of clarity about what is normal makes it more difficult to know what is abusive. They are left with a terrible legacy to resolve and understand, to try to bury, forget, and hide (Rosencrans, 1997). They are left with a profound sense that something is drastically wrong with them, that they are deeply disturbed and perverse.

Just as they were silenced in childhood, mother-daughter incest survivors are muted in their adult lives. Once again, the wounded child within is silenced, this time by a society that continues to deny that mothers do sexually abuse their daughters. The child, and later the adult, cannot reveal those awful things that were done to her by her mother, for fear of exposing her innate badness or revealing that she is tainted, depraved, and damaged goods. She perceives herself as evil, unloved, and unwanted. These perceptions are as acute as the fear of being "found out." As adults, the central organizing principle is secrecy, which perpetuates the shame of childhood. Shame keeps the child and the adult survivor of mother-daughter incest silent, shrouded in secrecy, and trapped in a world of rejection, isolation, and stigmatization.

Mother-daughter incest survivors remain invisible because their trauma is not easily identified. They go unnoticed by practitioners who are unable to hear that a woman might abuse. Mother-daughter incest survivors often feel silenced and betrayed by the helping practitioners who are willing to hear that a father can be incestuous but will not recognize or hear clues that a mother could be sexually abusive to her daughter. When they decide to break their silence, often their disclosures are met with revulsion and condemnation. Often, they will not reveal their secret.

Incestuous behavior by abusive mothers will continue to go unnoticed, underreported, and underinvestigated as long as society buries its head in ignorance. Society will remain an active part of the conspiracy, and silence will remain the greatest barrier to recovery for the mother-daughter incest survivor. As long as society evades the truth that mother-daughter incest does happen, the consequences of this form of victimization will remain hidden and so will its profound implications that extend far and deep in the lives of its survivors.

## THE WOMEN IN THIS STUDY

Sixty-two adult female survivors of maternal sexual abuse from across the country were personally interviewed by the author about their abuse experiences. They were recruited through notices placed in women's centers, counseling offices, newspaper articles, radio talk shows, and by word of mouth. The women ranged in age from nineteen to fifty-six (average age thirty-nine), experienced an average of 11.5 years of sexual abuse by their mothers (range one to forty years), that began at the average age of 3.6 years (range six months to twelve years). Eight of the women were aboriginal, ten of European descent, and forty-four were Caucasian. Ninety percent of the women (fifty-six out of sixty-two) reported physical abuse as well as sexual abuse by their mothers, twenty-five of them (40.3 percent) described substance abuse in the home, and 22 (35 percent) of them narrated sexual abuse by their father or stepfather as well. Twenty-four (39 percent) of the women recounted that one or more of their siblings were also sexually abused by their mother. These women were in therapy an average of ten years (range one to twenty-eight years). Twenty (32 percent) of the women are mothers themselves, thirty-nine are single, four separated, ten divorced, and nine married. Thirty-six communicated that they came from middle-class families, twelve from upper middle-class families, and fourteen from lower class families. Thirteen of the women graduated from high school, ten dropped out of school, twelve received postsecondary or undergraduate degrees, ten attained graduate degrees, and two received their doctorates. Nineteen of the women disclosed that they were the eldest child, eighteen the youngest child, eight the middle child, and eleven the only child.

# Chapter 2

# The Essential Human Connection

Many authors have theoretically addressed the significance of the mother-daughter relationship. An exploration of the uniqueness of the mother-daughter relationship provides a context in which the impact of mother-daughter incest may be better understood. Developmental theory and attachment theory can be applied to the exploration of the uniqueness of the mother-daughter relationship. Furthermore, these theories provide a context in which the repercussions of mother-daughter incest may be better understood.

The mother-child bond has been called the essential human connection, one that teaches us how to love and without which we cannot be whole human beings. A mother's love provides basic security, stability, nurturing admiration (a general feeling of individual worth), warmth and physical affection, cuddling, holding and kissing, caring, and acceptance. We receive courage, sense of self, the ability to believe we have value as human beings, and the ability to love others as well as ourselves, from the strength of our mother's love for us when we are infants. As our first mirror of life, mother functions as protector, guide, and interpreter.

A unique tie exists between mother and daughter in our society which is encouraged and supported through societal values. A young girl's identification with her mother continues throughout life, thereby maintaining the mother-daughter relationship while establishing her identity. As women, society encourages us to carry our mothers with us in every breath, every decision, every success, and every failure. Our sense of self as a daughter is entwined with a sense of mother. We look to our mothers in terms of how we define ourselves, in terms of what it is to be a woman and what it is to be a daughter. In essence, there is a shared social role, a shared prescription for life, and a shared psychology. The inevitable modeling relationship between mother and daughter leaves the image of her as a woman, with a sense of basic trust that her mother gave her. Tender, but many times painful, lessons learned from mother in the way she loved us, and the way she loved herself, stay with us for life.

Society expects mothers to feel the need to continue their role as mothers since it has been an integral part of their female identity and of how they have defined themselves in the world. Cultural bias demands that mothers keep their daughters tied to them. Through maintaining attachments with their daughters, mothers are encouraged to fulfill their needs for interpersonal connectedness, for relatedness. Society gives mothers more license to hold onto their daughters and mother them, to become gratified yet fearful as they witness their daughters move forward in a positive and competent manner.

## *DEVELOPMENTAL THEORY*

Many authors (Flax, 1989; LaSorsa and Fodor, 1990; Stiver, 1991; Boyd, 1989) have addressed the notion of the mutuality of the mother-daughter relationship. Genuine mother-daughter love has been described as a recognition on the part of each of the separateness of the other and a respect for the other. A true loving mother has interest and happiness in seeing her daughter as a person, not just a possession. She is generous and loving to such an extent that she forgoes some of her own pleasure and security to add to her daughter's development.

As with attachment theorists, developmentalists address stages of achievement of mother and daughter that are obtained through the mother's ability to anticipate and respond to the child's reaching out for growth. For the relationship between mother and daughter to proceed harmoniously, each must be aware of the other's viewpoints, goals, feelings, and intentions. Each must adjust her own behavior to align with the other. This requires that each has reasonably accurate models of self and other which are regularly updated and negotiated by full communication between them. These interchanges go on throughout life, forming a complex pattern of mutuality. Each developmental stage requires of them the ability to lose their ties and maintain their connections.

The mother-daughter bond has been identified as complex, unique, and emotionally charged. Although described as one of the strongest bonds throughout life, it has also been described as more ambivalent and ambiguous than other parent-child dyads. Developmentalists tend to describe the mother-daughter relationship in terms of life cycle categories or stages: symbiosis, separation, and individuation. They highlight the mutuality of the mother-daughter relationship with its intense needs flowing in both directions, which must give way to separateness as the daughter struggles to be her own person. The struggle for independence is in eternal conflict with this symbiotic bond and the will toward oneness.

During the first three years of human life, the most important developmental tasks are establishing a close relationship with mother and then moving or separating from that relationship through the process of *individuation*. The symbiotic bond, which is developed during the first six or seven months of life, provides the grounding on which the infant can rely as it moves out of the symbiotic orbit into differentiation and exploration of the outside world. The omnipotent system, this dual unity within one boundary system of ontological security for the infant, eventually gives way to a developmental track which sees the child take pleasure in his or her own developing capacities. *Separation* involves the establishment of a firm sense of differentiation from the mother, of possessing one's own physical and mental boundaries. The individuation process will see the development of a range of characteristics, skills, and personality traits that are uniquely one's own. Ideally, the relationship is able to negotiate an appropriate middle ground between dependency and isolation. Rather than a relationship which swings from one pole of the continuum to the other, a healthy balanced position is achieved, one of appropriate interdependence.

Differentiation overlaps with the *practicing phase* (Flax, 1989) from ten to eighteen months when the child develops pleasure in its own locomotor skills and a rudimentary autonomous ego. The child will find it difficult to develop his or her capacities if the mother is ambivalent about giving up the symbiotic phase or if she is parasitic (reliving her own infancy through the child). This is more likely to be true for the female child.

The third developmental phase of separation-individuation, called the *rapprochement phase,* occurs when the child is approximately fifteen to twenty-four months of age. This stage is characterized by ambivalence. The child wants to return to the symbiotic state yet fears being reengulfed by it. Fear of losing the love of the mother becomes increasingly evident. Girls seem to be more engrossed with their mothers' presence and demand a greater closeness. On the other hand, the mother may experience her own ambivalence about her adult role during this period. The fact that society highly endorses this symbiosis between mother and daughter complicates this process, making it difficult to break through. Mother and daughter are persistently enmeshed in the ambivalent aspects of the relationship, which is viewed by society as a sticky, gooey closeness and some idyllic, wonderful experience. Ambivalence may characterize the mother-daughter relationship more than any other relationship in human life.

Developmentally, separation and individuation, or self-definition, become the two main tasks of adolescence. Adolescence has been described in the literature as the most difficult period for the mother-daughter dyad because of the tremendous anxiety that occurs between them. Both the adolescent daughter and the midlife mother face the developmental challenges of separation, autonomy, and loss, as well as the need for a new definition of self. Although daughters during this adolescent period are often rebelliously striving to free themselves from the old bonds of childhood—from mother's apron strings, so to speak—they often still consider their mother as their confidante, as the person to whom they feel closest. The strong mother-daughter bond that developed from a very young age and has continued over the years makes separation a painful and arduous task for both.

It is not surprising, then, that developmentalists have historically characterized the mother-daughter relationship as a process of holding on and letting go, of maintaining an ongoing attachment as they begin to separate. Nor is it surprising that some mothers, as they witness their daughters developing strong needs for privacy and making others their confidantes, find this separation extremely painful. Some mothers may not understand their daughters' needs to establish separate spaces for themselves. They may possess their children out of loneliness, fear of failure, and need of confirmation of womanliness in their world. They may not let go of their daughters because they have little else in their lives or nothing of their own. They may have been so frustrated in their relationships with their own mothers that they try to make up for it through symbiosis with their daughters.

They may be trying to fill up the empty hole left inside by their own cold, distant, or absent mother. Merging with their daughters and wanting them to be the other half of them may provide the warm extension for which they have longed. It may replace what they never had with their own mothers. When this happens, the daughter is given little latitude and little chance for growth.

## OBJECT-RELATIONS THEORY

Object-relations theory provides an often-cited framework for examining the mother-daughter dyad, a framework based on traditional psychoanalytic and social thought. Drawing on object-relations theory, Chodorow (1974, 1978) speculates that societal values which encourage and support the early attachment of mother and daughter, allow for self-other boundary flexibility in girls. Chodorow shows an interest in identity formation as it pertains to issues concerning attachment, association, and separation. She acknowledges that less social pressure is placed on daughters to differentiate from their mothers than on sons to differentiate from their fathers. Boys, in contrast, are socially supported to curtail the primary identification with mother. Chodorow concedes that the mother-daughter same-gender relationship is characterized by boundaries that are less clearly defined than for mothers and sons. As a result, less effort is required for boys to establish their identity.

The more contemporary object-relations theorists, such as LaSorsa and Fodor (1990) emphasize that for adolescent girls, the process of separation-individuation is made more complex, unique, and emotionally charged than other parent-child dyads because of the longer and more intense identification between mother and daughter in the daughter's early years. They warn that loose boundaries and a less separate sense of self are likely to cause mothers and daughters to grapple with the development of separate identities. Greater effort is required of adolescent girls to achieve autonomy and separateness. Conflicts over the need to separate are thought to arise from a perceived lack of psychological distance within the dyad.

## *SELF-IN-RELATION (RELATIONAL) THEORY*

Self-in-relation, an evolving theory of women's development postulated by Miller (1976), Gilligan (1982), and Surrey (1985) and developed by Jordan and Surrey (1986), Stiver (1991), and Kaplan (1991), puts forth a new model of female development and identity based on a reinterpretation of current psychoanalytic theory and a search for principles of self-development, keeping in mind that women's reality is different from men's. Rather than focusing on separation, this more recent perspective emphasizes attachment and connecting as the basis for female identity development. The focus is on relationship differentiation rather than separation-individuation. Differentiation is viewed as a dynamic process of growth within the relationship in which women organize their sense of identity, find existential meaning, and achieve a sense of coherence and continuity and are motivated in the context of a relationship.

Self-in-relation theory involves an important shift in emphasis from separation to relationships as the basis for development. For women, the primary experience of self is relational; the self unfolds in the context of important relationships (Boyd, 1989). The development of the core relational self for women is initiated by the dynamic of the early mother-child relationship. This dynamic is characterized by finely tuned affected sensitivity, availability, and responsiveness of the mother to the daughter, and vice versa. Healthy mother-daughter interactions are based on connectedness, on open physical and emotional sharing, as well as on early mutuality of caring. Aspects of self-development such as creativity, autonomy, and assertion emerge in the context of relationship. There is no ingrained need to disconnect or to sacrifice relationship for self-development.

For self-in-relation theorists, the open relationship between mother and daughter with flexible self-boundaries intensifies empathic sensitivity in females (Stiver, 1991; Kaplan, 1991). The mother-daughter dyad is the beginning stage for the development of self-in-relation in which the mutual sharing process fosters a sense of mutual understanding and connection. This is the motivational dynamic of mutual improvement that leaves both mother and daughter mobilized to care for and attend to the well-being and development of the other. This two-way interactional model involves a process of growth within relationship in which both are encouraged and challenged to maintain connection and to foster, adapt to, and change the growth of the other. Identity is based, then, on positive association.

For the mother-daughter incest survivor, the basic components of a mother's love are nonexistent. A relationship characterized by mutuality and sensitivity has not been fostered. Over time the reciprocal process, in which mother and daughter become highly responsive to the feelings of each other, has not developed. Conditions have not fostered the unique tie between mother and daughter in which both are energized to care for and respond to the well-being of the other.

Survivors of mother-daughter incest have no capacity to be attuned to the affect of others, to understand and be understood by another, and to participate in the development of others. The daughter does not experience the well-being of the mother-daughter relationship as a source for self-esteem and self-affirmation. She does not savor the flow of empathic communication and mutual attentiveness from one to the other. She is not permitted to feel that she is cared for. A sense of herself as a caring being, as one who derives strength and competence from her own relational capacities, cannot be allowed to evolve. In short, her reason to be, her primary motivational thrust, her core relational self, her self-structure, has been denied.

When a child or adult is prevented from participating in mutually enhancing relationships, a sense of disconnection occurs. For the mother-daughter incest survivor, as for victims of other forms of abuse, this disconnection occurs because, as a child, she was grossly abused and her surrounding relational context was insensitive to the expression of her experience. One might argue that our society collectively remains insensitive to the mother-daughter incest survivor's expression of her experience, even when as an adult she attempts to break her silence.

A mother-daughter incest survivor has been denied her essential connection. She was not nurtured or reared with warmth, caring, and guidance. She has been party to the most disturbed expression of maladaptivity of any mothering role. Essentially, she has experienced the most extreme disconnection and violation because she was sexually abused. Because she was violated physically and sexually by the one person in the world who was supposed to protect, nurture, and guide her, this violence is reprehensible and representative of the most severe form of psychological violation and detachment. This violation is exacerbated because she has been disallowed, disempowered, and denied opportunity to tell the truth about her experience. When the mother is the perpetrator, the profound betrayal of trust and the taboo and enforced silence surrounding the phenomenon profoundly contribute to the deep wounding and the devastating impact on the daughter's life.

## ATTACHMENT THEORY

Attachment theory emphasizes the powerful influence on a child's development of the way he or she is treated by his or her parents, especially the mother. Attachment behavior is any form of behavior that results in a person attaining or maintaining proximity to some other clearly identified individual who is perceived as better able to cope with the world. Attachment researchers address the notion of using the parent as a secure base from which the child explores the world. The mother usually provides this secure base since she is often the primary caregiver. Infants need to know that their primary caregiver is reliable and dependable. Knowing that an attachment figure is accessible, available, and responsive gives an individual a strong and pervasive feeling of security. It encourages the individual to value and continue the relationship. Fortified with the knowledge that his or her mother is there and available, the child is able to go forth to explore the world, learn about it, and acquire the skills to master what is encountered along the way. The infant essentially is liberated and becomes autonomous by the mother's warm, sensitive care. Connected mothers enable their children to feel valued in a positive world, to feel confident enough to explore, to develop healthy relationships, and to rebound from adversity.

## ATTACHMENT BEHAVIORS

Bowlby (1988) defined a series of developmental stages based on the maternal bond, which have real implications when exploring the mother-daughter bond. During the first year of a child's existence, he or she is gradually able to display a range of *attachment behaviors,* disapproving and protesting his or her mother's departure, greeting her upon her return, clinging to her when frightened, and following her when able. Such actions are rooted in the biological fact that proximity to the mother is satisfying and essential to survival. It is the establishment, maintenance, and ongoing renewal of this proximity that begets feelings of love, security, and connection. A disruption of this joy, especially if it is lasting or untimely, often brings about anxiety, grief, sadness, and even depression for the child.

Infants, then, have built-in needs for relatedness, and develop unconscious working models of self and other, partially reflective of how well their mothers respond and tend to these needs. Secure attachment in early childhood is a principal factor in predicting healthy functioning in teenage and adult years. The pattern of attachment that an individual develops during the years of immaturity, notably infancy, childhood, and adolescence, is profoundly influenced by the way parents or other parent figures treat the child. The parent-child relationship, and more particularly the mother-child interaction, is known to be extremely important for the child's mental and emotional growth. Children who have sensitive and responsive parents are enabled to develop along healthy pathways. Children who have insensitive, unresponsive, neglectful, or rejecting parents are likely to develop along deviant pathways that are incompatible with good mental health and which renders them vulnerable to breakdown, should they meet with seriously adverse effects.

This concept of a secure personal base from which a child, adolescent, or adult goes out to explore, and to which the individual returns from time to time, provides insight into how emotional stability develops and functions over the life span. The capacity to make emotional bonds with other individuals, whether in a care-seeking role or a caregiving role, is regarded as a predominant characteristic of effective personality functioning and mental health. A person's mental state is deeply influenced by whether relationships are warm and harmonious or tense, angry, and anxious.

A child bonds with parents who are looked to for protection, comfort, and assistance. The model they build for themselves is a reflection of the images that their parents have of them. These images are communicated not only by how each parent treats the child but also by what each says to the child. A child's self-model is profoundly influenced by how the child's mother sees and treats him or her. A securely attached individual has developed through continuous monitoring by the caregiver. When children signal that they want attention, their mothers register these signals and respond accordingly.

According to Bowlby (1988), a pathogenic family situation can be easily understood in terms of attachment theory. A mother may have grown up *insecurely* attached as a result of a difficult childhood. She may burden her own daughter with expectations that she care for her, thus inverting the normal relationship of care-seeking attached child to caregiving parent. Many mother-daughter incest survivors, due to adverse experiences during childhood, have grown up to be over-involved and overly dependent on others and therefore more prone to seek care from their own children. If the mother in childhood suffered neglect and frequent severe threats of abandonment or physical assault, she is more prone than others to abuse her own child physically, resulting in adverse effects on her child's developing personality.

A second pattern of attachment is *anxious resistant attachment* in which the individual is uncertain whether a parent will be available, responsive, or helpful when called upon. Because of this uncertainty, the individual is always prone to separation anxiety, tends to be clingy, and is anxious about exploring the world. This pattern, in which conflict is evident, is promoted by a parent being available and helpful on some occasions but not on others, and by separations and, as clinical findings show, threats of abandonment used as a means of control.

*Anxious avoidant attachment* is a third pattern of attachment in which the individual has no confidence that when she seeks care, she will be responded to helpfully by the caregiver. On the contrary, she expects to be rebuffed. When, in marked degree, the individual attempts to live her life without the love and support of others, she tries to become emotionally self-sufficient and may later be diagnosed as narcissistic or as having a false self. This pattern, in which conflict is more hidden, is the result of the individual's mother constantly rebuffing her when she approaches her for comfort or protection. In contrast to securely attached infants, the anxiously attached child has not had her state consistently monitored but has instead had only sporadic monitoring. All too often, responses from mother are tardy or inappropriate. Avoidant children engage in direct communication only when they are content. The most extreme cases result from repeated rejections. This pattern may be shown by infants of mothers who are still preoccupied with mourning a parental figure lost during the mother's childhood and by those mothers who themselves suffered physical or sexual abuse as children.

Because of their own unresolved attachment issues, mothers whose needs were poorly met by their parents are at considerably greater risk to provide the sensitive caregiving needed by infants. When great stress is experienced by the mother during the critical period for attachment (conditions such as poverty, poor housing, nonsupporting partner, or psychological factors) and few supports are available to counteract this stress, the infant's capacity for attachment is at risk. Some mothers may be so damaged by their own life experiences that they are incapable or unable to provide sustained, sensitive attention and nurturing that infants require for optimal growth and development. The child's capacity to attach, to self-regulate, and to develop cognitively will be undermined if she is part of a neglectful or abusive family.

A mother who fails to respond in a helpful manner when her child is in distress and who repeatedly and impatiently rejects her child, leaves the child feeling suspicious of everyone else. While the child constantly yearns for the love and care she never receives, she has no confidence that she will ever receive it. She may need to express all her grief and unspeakable anguish for herself as a cast-off child (Bowlby, 1988). Small wonder, therefore, that when a woman with this background becomes a mother, there are times when instead of being ready to mother her child, she looks to her child to mother her. Small wonder, too, that when her child fails to oblige and starts crying, demanding care and attention, the mother becomes impatient and angry. It is against this background that a mother's violent assaults on a child can be understood.

When looking at the effects on personality development of mother-daughter incest survivors who were victimized as children, we must bear in mind that these women had no essential human connection or secure attachment to their mothers. Children suffer grievously and perhaps irreparably because this attachment to a primary caregiver was interrupted or lost. A secure home base conducive to optimal functioning and good mental health was denied the child because the mother was not readily available, sensitive to her child's signals, and lovingly responsive when the child needed protection and comfort. For the mother-daughter incest survivor, physical and sexual assaults are not the only episodes of antipathy from the mother. In many cases, these assaults represent the tip of the iceberg; they are usually manifestations of repeated episodes of prolonged angry rejection.

The psychological effects can be regarded as the outcome of enduring hostile rejection and neglect.

## APPLYING ATTACHMENT THEORY
## IN THE CLIENT-THERAPIST RELATIONSHIP

The practitioner must understand that caregiving, the major role of parents that is complementary to attachment behavior, is regarded in the same light as careseeking, namely as a basic component of human nature. A variation in the way the bond between parent and child develops and becomes organized during infancy and childhood is a huge determinant of whether a person grows up to be mentally healthy. When a mother is sexually abusive to her daughter, the relationship is characterized by the most severe form of physical and psychological disconnection and violation. When mother is the perpetrator, empathic communication and mutual attentiveness are absent, robbing the child of self-esteem and self-affirmation.

The therapist applying attachment theory sees his or her role as being one of providing the conditions in which the client can explore her representational models of herself and her attachment figures. In therapy, the mother-daughter incest survivor can appraise and restructure them in the light of the new understanding she acquires and the new experiences she has in the therapeutic relationship. The therapist will need to provide a secure base from which the mother-daughter incest survivor can explore the various unhappy and painful aspects of her life, past and present. The therapist as a trusted companion provides support, encouragement, empathy, and guidance. He or she can assist the client in her explorations by encouraging her to examine the ways she engages in relationships with significant others in her current life. She can explore her expectations for her own feelings and behavior and for those of other people as well. The therapist can encourage examination of the client-therapist relationship. The client is likely to import her perceptions and constructions of how an attachment figure is expected to behave and feel into the therapeutic alliance.

The client will need to consider how her current perceptions, expectations, actions, and feelings may be the product of the events she has encountered during childhood and adolescence, especially those situations with her parents. The therapist must be aware that this may be a painful and difficult process for the client since it involves look-ing at feelings about her parents, in particular her mother, that are un-imaginable and unthinkable. The client may be moved by strong emotions and urges to action, some of which may be directed toward her parents, and some toward the therapist. She may find many of these thoughts and emotions frightening, alien, and unacceptable.

The therapist needs to be aware that mother-daughter incest survi-vors may be attachment resistant during childhood, adolescence, and even adulthood. The survivor may tend to distance herself from the therapist, making the formation of the therapeutic alliance unlikely. Therapy that is reality based may help the mother-daughter incest survivor to identify and validate her feelings and to express them in ways less likely to repeat the past by evoking rejection and abuse from others. A goal of therapy should be to help the mother-daughter incest survivor learn to recognize and give voice to her feelings in-stead of acting out those feelings.

The therapist also has the task of enabling the client to recognize that her images of herself and others, many of them derived from past painful experiences or from a parent, may not be appropriate for her present and future. The therapist can encourage her to grasp the na-ture of her governing images or models, trace their beginnings, and begin to understand what has conditioned her to think, feel, and act in a particular manner. Only then is she in the position to reflect on the accuracy and adequacy of these images in light of her current experi-ences and relationships with emotionally significant people in her life, including herself. She will see the old images for what they are and feel free to imagine and pursue a preferred scenario of alterna-tives that are a better fit for her current life. The therapist, then, en-ables his or her client to cease being a slave to old and unconscious stereotypes and to feel, think, and act in new ways.

The therapist's role is to provide a secure base from which the cli-ent can express her thoughts and feelings. This is analogous to the role of a mother to provide a secure base from which to explore the world. The therapist strives to be reliable, attentive, and empathic in his or her responses to the client's explorations. At the same time, the therapist understands that the client may not trust him or her. The therapist needs to provide the care for and attention that the client yearns for. The therapist needs to be aware of his or her own contribu-tion to the therapeutic process, to his or her relationship to the client that reflects to a certain extent the therapist's childhood experiences. The focus in therapy can be the here and now, on the interactions between the client and the therapist.

Finally, the client may be expecting the therapist to reject, criticize, or humiliate her. An anxiously avoidant client may behave in a manner of emotional self-containment and insulation against intimate contacts with other people. She may seem narcissistic or have a false self. She may avoid therapy and keep the therapist at arm's length. The therapist will require a prolonged, quiet, and friendly patience. The client may experience the terror of being subjected to something similar from the therapist as the constant rebuffing by her mother when she was a child. She may fear that the therapist will try to trap her into a relationship aimed to serve the therapist's interests, a fear originating in childhood when her mother made her an attachment figure and caregiver. Chapters 17 and 18 of this book further explore transferencial-countertransferencial dynamics between client and therapist and their effects on the process and outcomes of therapy.

# PART II:
# COMMON THEMES
# AMONG DAUGHTERS

The data analysis of the in-depth personal interviews with the women about their experience of sexual abuse at the hands of their mothers yielded the following common salient themes:

1. Acute shame
2. Trapped with no place to go
3. Double-crossed: betrayal and grief
4. Identification with and differentiation from mother
5. Impaired sexual development
6. Difficulty coping

Each theme deserves its own chapter which includes suggestions for therapeutic practice and treatment recommendations.

# Chapter 3

# Acute Shame

I still think I was a bad kid. I'm not past the shame yet. I really don't want people to know what happened. It's hard for me to say that I am a mother-daughter incest survivor. There's always been this weird feeling. It's very isolating because it's not something I want to talk about. It's such a taboo subject.

*Jan*

As a result of analyzing the dynamics of child sexual abuse, Finkelhor and Browne (1985) postulated that the following four factors are most related to traumatization in the victim:

1. *Traumatic sexualization*—A process in which a child's sexuality is shaped in a developmentally inappropriate and interpersonally dysfunctional fashion as a result of the sexual abuse
2. *Betrayal*—The dynamic by which children discover that someone on whom they were dependent caused them harm
3. *Powerlessness*—The process in which the child's will, desires, and sense of efficacy are continually contravened
4. *Stigmatization*—The negative connotations (e.g., badness, shame, and guilt) which are communicated to the child regarding the experience and which then become incorporated into the child's self-image

The conjunction of these four dynamics in the sexual abuse experience makes the trauma of sexual abuse unique.

This model can be utilized to demonstrate the extreme degree of trauma experienced by a mother-daughter incest victim. Certainly, mother-daughter incest victims lost their sexual innocence as children and had their sexuality shaped inappropriately and prematurely as a result of their traumatic sexual abuse. They experienced profound betrayal of trust due to the fact that they were harmed as children by someone upon whom they had been vitally dependent. They felt powerless when their will, desires, and sense of efficacy were continually contravened. They were forced, threatened, coerced, or deceived to submit to unwanted sexual acts. They felt powerless to end the abuse. Stigma occurred when their deep secrets caused them to fear blame for the adult's actions and rejection by the world around them. Negative messages were communicated to these women when they were children and these messages eventually became integrated into their self-images. At the same time, they were undergoing socialization by a society that idealizes motherhood and ostracizes homosexuals. This served to ensure their silence and cause them additional shame, fear, and concern.

These women as children were compelled to participate in sexual experiences that were confusing to them. They felt profoundly betrayed by the one person they trusted the most and by a society that forced their silence. Powerless to stop any of it and ashamed to their very core, the trauma they experienced was intensified, and their development throughout childhood, adolescence, and adulthood was hindered. They sustained severe physical, emotional, and psychological damage that resulted in long-lasting scarring.

> I certainly was brutally penetrated by men at a very young age. Yet the emotional impact of having to perform this sexual act with my mother is just so devastating. The issues just feel so much more complex. There are a lot of similarities but the shame, the stigma, the isolation that come out of being abused by your mother, make it so difficult to talk about. What brought me to the crux of writing that letter to Mother was I thought I was going to die. When the memories and the grief came up, and the intensity of the betrayal, I thought I was going to die. I thought, *I am going to die from this.* In fact I wanted to die. I made plans but then I thought, *Hey, kid, it's you or your mother. Who are you going to pick?* I decided I was worth it and it was going to be her to die, not me. I was going to take the risk actually knowing full well that as soon as I put the letter in the

mail, this could be it, but you can live. You're strong enough now to live with whatever comes out of this, even losing your mother.

*Mable*

She is shamed by what she *is;* she feels soiled and spoiled, contaminated to her inner core by the dirty reprehensible act of incest. The mother-daughter incest survivor, because of the strength of her connection with her mother, feels that she asked for the abuse or permitted it to happen.

> Simply by virtue of her existence on earth, she believes that she has driven the most powerful person in her world to do terrible things. Surely then her nature must be thoroughly evil. Her language of her self becomes the language of abomination. (Herman, 1992, p. 105)

As a developing child, these feelings of being damaged to the core were etched into the very fabric of her being. Her sense of inner badness was ratified again and again by her mother's scapegoating. She was further shamed when she struggled with her anger, leaving her believing that she is a hateful person. She magnified her self-deprecation when she uncontrollably unloaded her anger and displaced it far from its dangerous source.

For many mother-daughter incest survivors, shame colors everything they think or feel and how they interact with others. They are often left with low self-image, with self-loathing, and with self-hate. They may try to be perfect or the best at everything, but underneath they feel ugly, defective, stupid, and absolutely evil. Even as adults, they feel vulnerable and unlovable. The little girl in them is profoundly wounded and traumatized.

Many mother-daughter incest survivors will express in the therapeutic process that they feel responsible for their abuse, that they somehow caused, engineered, or contributed to what they term a distasteful, disturbing, degrading experience. Many of these women feel profound shame because their perception of their abuse experience is that they failed to resist it. They view themselves as the root of the problem and as having brought it on themselves. The practitioner needs to understand that the mother-daughter incest survivor believes she is basically defective as a human being. She believes she is flawed, smaller, or lower than others. She believes she is a shame, not just ashamed. The abuse and neglect at the hands of her mother have convinced her that she is bad because bad things happen only to bad people. The clinician needs to be cognizant that, as the victim gets older, her self-blame and shame may intensify, and she may forget her powerlessness as a child. The clinician must emphasize just how powerless the client was as a child to control the events in her life.

When it is impossible to avoid the reality of the abuse, the child must construct some system of meaning that justifies it. It is not uncommon for children who have been abused to try to make sense of what happened to them by preserving the belief that they can still trust the abuser. Especially if the perpetrator is a parent, children tell themselves that the abuse happened because they are innately bad. Inevitably, they conclude that if they are bad, then their parents are good. This sense of inner badness may gradually dissipate as the survivor increases awareness about the abuse and accepts the fact that he or she was manipulated and coerced by an older, more powerful abuser. As victims preserve a sense of meaning, hope, and power, they become convinced that if they brought this fate upon themselves, then they have the power to change it.

Although many mother-daughter incest survivors feel damaged to the core and powerless to stop feelings of being damaged, and as they spend their childhood and adulthood feeling dirty and ashamed, part of them may still hope that one day, someday, their mother will want them, will make it all better, and will make them feel special. The mother-daughter incest survivor believes that if she drove her mother to abuse her, then if she tries hard enough she may earn her mother's forgiveness and win the love and protection that she so desperately craves.

> There's such a push-pull thing. Wanting to get close to her, being pushed away and then thinking *the hell with this.* I would say to her, "Let's just you and I go out for a cup of coffee," and, "No, no, can't. Don't have time" But when I withdrew, there was still the dance going on and so that was very frustrating. I felt like a total failure and not knowing why. I guess I didn't know why she couldn't love me. If my own mother can't love me, then who the heck is going to? It's a belief that our mothers should love us, at

the very least. A good mother loves her children, I think, don't they? If my own mother doesn't love me, how can I love myself 'cause I've never learned how.

*Sonia*

The practitioner needs to understand that adult incest survivors who blame themselves often are more depressed, whereas those who blame their abuser are less depressed, have higher self-esteem, and have a high self-concept (Hoagwood, 1990). Internal attributions of self-blame may be more maladaptive for the mother-daughter incest survivor in that her recovery from the trauma may be poor. Low self-worth associated with self-blame has developed over the years for the mother-daughter incest survivor. These self-blame attributions may be more resistant to change for the mother-daughter incest survivor because she typically blames herself in two ways: *characterological self-blame* (e.g., "The abuse happened because I am a bad person") and *behavioral self-blame* (e.g., "The abuse happened because of what I did").

At age nine when my mother fondled my breasts, I remember feeling tremendous shame. I thought I had provoked her and somehow brought it on. I felt I was bad. I remember Mother pushing me against the wall and being rough. I felt physical pain yet sexual stimulation.

*Soulitsa*

Why is this happening to me and not them? I grew up thinking that I must have done something wrong for her to sexually abuse me, that it was me and whatever I was doing. I never could understand it but I always blamed myself for why I was being hurt all the time. She didn't do these things to my sister and brother. When they got in trouble, they didn't to the extent that I did. It wasn't the same. That is part of the shame that I feel. I knew there must be something wrong with me. It must be something I am doing.

*Val*

Chronic doubts about what did or did not happen, along with persistent inability to trust one's perception of reality, are perhaps the most permanent and ultimately damaging long-term effects of childhood sexual abuse (Davies and Frawley, 1994). The practitioner will need to be aware that the mother-daughter incest survivor, because she feels guilty and tainted, may bury her secret deep within her mind. She may desperately want to believe it never happened. She may reach a point where she believes that she must have imagined what happened to her—that it could not have really taken place. Her feeling that her perception of the abuse is somehow distorted serves to exacerbate her assumptions that her experience was just a fantasy and that she is crazy and evil. As an adult, she may find that carrying her deep-rooted shame is too overwhelming and that it is far easier to doubt her memories than to live with them or take the blame for her abuse experience.

> I guess it's the word incest—I choke over that one. I feel I have to apologize somehow. When I have disclosed to a few people that I was sexually abused by my mother I often got the comment back, "Are you sure? You really think so?" or I get this look of disgust on their face. I still take it personally as if somehow it's directed toward me and I'm to blame. You feel that the memories are wrong and especially in the beginning you really doubt them. You must have made a mistake and you're wrong. I decided to feel the doubt and carry on.
>
> *Sonia*

The helping professional will need to be aware that many mother-daughter incest survivors, like other abuse victims, feel such unbearable rage, shame, or fear that they may act self-abusively. Often the cycle is self-generating; when she hurts herself she feels disgusted with her behavior, and so punishes herself further through another round of self-harm. Her strongly held belief that she is bad, that she is to blame for the abuse, that she is incompetent, unlovable, and disgusting activates feelings of rage, fear, grief, and anxiety. These distressing feelings then trigger the self-injurious behavior (Miller, 1994). This powerful combination of pain, fear, and pleasure allows the victim to experience herself as "bad" through her feelings of shame, and so the cycle continues.

The clinician will need to be open to the fact that during the therapeutic process, self-blame and shame may take the form of self-criticism and condemnation by these women. Survivors of mother-daughter incest may define themselves as deficient individuals not only in their daughter role, but also in their role as mother to their own children. The mother-daughter incest survivor may need help to recognize her shame, label it, and express her feelings. The practitioner will need to remind her that it is not so much about who she is as it is about how she was parented and treated as a child. Improving the client's basic assumptions or beliefs about herself and the world may assist her in the resolution of her traumatic experience of sexual abuse at the hands of her mother (Ullman, 1997). The focus of therapy should be in building the survivor's positive view of herself or, in other words, strengthening her self-image regarding all of her positive attributes. She can be encouraged to think of herself in positive ways, and to perhaps purchase a book of affirmations for herself. She may benefit from an affirming letter written to herself that highlights her good points. When feeling down or shameful, she might read this letter to receive a boost. She will need to solicit the support of her closest friends in order to feel good about herself as a worthy individual.

The therapist needs to be receptive to the fact that the shame of mother-daughter incest is more profound and the stigmatizing more extreme because the abuse experience is in the minority and out of the ordinary. Hence, the mother-daughter incest survivor may feel more reluctant to disclose that her mother was her abuser. She may even allow her therapist or group members to assume that her abuse was male perpetrated, perhaps by her father. Intense feelings of shame may be expressed by mother-daughter incest survivors in the form of discomfort with their bodies. They are often uncomfortable with the physical features that they feel resemble their mothers. They may despise looking like their mothers in any way and may go to great lengths to alter their appearance, or cover it up, to look different from their mothers. They may resent their femininity because it connects them to their mother. They may show disgust with their bodies, in particular with their genitals, because their mothers took great pleasure from them or coerced the daughters to perform specific sexual acts. Some women literally hate their bodies as a result of the abuse. They may feel that their bodies betrayed them or let them down, especially if they were sexually stimulated or orgasmic during the abuse experience. Perhaps these women were left to feel that they had no control over their bodies during their abuse experience, which may contribute to their feelings of self-blame and shame, even self-hatred. Participation in forbidden sexual activity also confirms for the mother-daughter incest survivor her sense of inner badness. If she experienced sexual pleasure, enjoyed special attention from her mother, and/or bargained for favors or privileges, then these sins in her mind are indicative of her instigation and ultimate responsibility for the abuse and that she is innately wicked.

> I still blame myself for the abuse. I just figured that there must be something really wrong with me, that somehow it was my body . . . it's so hard not to believe it wasn't your fault when it's your mom who perpetrates against you.
> I hated my body from then on. I wore bathrobes and I tried to hide my body as much as possible. I still can't stand to look at my body. I'm so ashamed. I still dress in layers and I can't wear skimpy clothes. I'm afraid to go out in a bathing suit.

*Christine*

In summary, the mother-daughter incest survivor encounters a spiritual crisis at her very core. She feels hollowed out, subhuman, different from the rest of the world, and isolated from all the external sources of comfort. She feels that something about her is unacceptable which sets her apart. Acute shame threatens her core identity. Shame for the mother-daughter incest survivor may be associated with self-neglect, self-abuse, and self-sabotage. Self-harm can serve to express and release the grief that has been stored from the past and the grief that the mother-daughter incest survivor continues to experience in the present. The practitioner must be cognizant that the mother-daughter incest survivor may carry her own unexplored shame and self-hatred that may be expressed in the repetition of the abuse against her own daughter. She may re-enact her own abuse by harming herself, or less often, by abusing her own children.

Clinically, the survivor will need ongoing assistance to heal the wounds of shame. The process of acceptance for the survivor of her powerlessness as a child and of casting off her guilt and self-blame may be arduous. Upon acceptance, she can start the process of doing something for herself once she starts being completely honest about the abuse and its effects on her. Part of this acceptance involves the realization that the abuser was responsible for the abuse and that the survivor can take back her power as she becomes responsible for her recovery.

Therapy may provide the arena for mother-daughter incest survivors to build their self-esteem, recognize their strengths which enabled them to survive their abuse experience, confront guilt and self-blame, and break down feelings of isolation and shame. The clinician must allow the survivor to process her multiple losses and break away from patterns of behavior. Therapy may offer the survivor hope for a fuller, richer life—one void of feelings of fear and guilt.

It may be necessary for the therapist working with mother-daughter incest survivors to reframe accepting help as an act of courage. The mother-daughter incest survivor will need to acknowledge the reality of her experience and that taking steps to change it are signs of strength, not weakness, initiative, not passivity. Taking action to foster recovery, far from granting victory to the perpetrator, empowers the survivor. The therapist may need to state this view explicitly and in detail in order to address the feelings of shame and defeat that all too often prevent the mother-daughter incest survivor from seeking help (Brassell, 1994).

# Chapter 4

# Trapped with No Place to Go

She was very controlling, very manipulative. She ruled like a dictator. Hell, she was Caesar! Sometimes I used to get her really pissed off and I'd say to her, "Heil, Hitler." When I got into high school and learned about this man, I thought, *Oh my God, he must be related to my mother.* I remember going home and saying "Heil, Hitler" to her one day and I just about died for that remark. She just about beat the living daylights out of me for that one.

*Iris*

Isolation is one of the most painful parts of any incest experience. The mother-daughter incest survivor's isolation is cultivated by the perpetrator's attempts to control and manipulate her. Mother-daughter incest survivors feel cut off from the outside world, isolated and alienated from possible sources of support and validation. They may feel that their world has crumbled away. They feel suppressed, dominated, or possessed by their mothers, who verbally and emotionally abused them, leaving them feeling worthless and powerless to stop the abuse. The combined issues of dominance, fear of loss, and secrecy made escape from their incestuous mothers unlikely for these women.

She'd get really violent and she'd try to kill me or kill herself. She would get really lucid. I would sometimes be able to reach her in some way and it felt like I could stop her. But the price I would have to pay for it was that I would promise her that I would do anything she wanted me to and that I really loved her. We would play this scenario out several times. I felt really tied to that because I felt if I didn't do what she wanted, she would kill herself.

*Mable*

The perpetrators' control over their victims actively reinforces the daughters' sense of being different from other people. These debilitating feelings of powerlessness prevent mother-daughter incest survivors from venturing outside the family and seeking help, support, or validation. The stigmatization they feel contributes to their silence regarding the abuse and cultivates their feelings of powerlessness to end the abuse. This nurtures in them a sense of aloneness and of being different.

> She would manipulate and control through words, through actions, through anger, through physical violence. That was her way. She attacked me with a knife and my father as well. She would attempt suicide or run away almost every week.
>
> *Alana*

Trapped with no place to go, mother-daughter incest survivors believe that they cannot reveal the truth about their abuse experience for fear of being further alienated. They feel, perhaps to a greater degree than survivors of other forms of sexual abuse, that they have no choice but to remain silent about their abuse, and that the isolation and secrecy regarding their abuse experience has been imposed on them.

Mother-daughter incest survivors keep their stories deeply concealed for many years even from their own consciousness. Hence a sense of helplessness and hopelessness is fostered in the minds of mother-daughter incest survivors. In their minds, disclosing that their mothers rejected them, abused them, or wished that they had not been born, would hold them suspect. They cannot risk being doubted by the world. They may try to ignore the existence of abuse out of fear of the consequences of speaking out.

It is not surprising, then, that mother-daughter incest survivors are often consummate actresses. They appear to be successful in the world, are often accomplished in the business world or the professional arena; many get married, and maintain relationships with friends and families. To the outside world, they seem to be average, well-adjusted adults, but inside they feel incredibly vulnerable, that the roof could cave in on them at any moment. In essence, they feel forced to carry their awful secret and intense unresolved feelings to their grave. Feeling trapped by their silence yet protected by it, they may lie and make excuses as to why they do not feel connected to their mothers or get along with them.

It is important for the practitioner to recognize the deep sense of confusion that a mother-daughter survivor feels about what is wrong with her. She may be a high achiever and a perfectionist but at the same time she is secretly aware of her deep hidden depression, her sense of despair, and a deep exhaustion that she may not understand. She may feel cut off from her feelings and her body. She feels guilt-ridden, different from others, and isolated. She desperately wants to believe that abuse at the hands of her mother never happened.

> I'm quite open about it and I am well accepted in my world of work. I have demonstrated to them how successful I am in working through it, and how I have continued on with my life. I'm pretty proud of myself for living through it all. I'm well respected in the community, and have a broader focus in life. I've improved my relationships. Admitting it to myself, I still like to escape it and believe it didn't happen. But my life has been telltale. I accept it as something I've conquered. I feel successful that way. I'm grateful for everybody that really helped, that they didn't give up on me and that I'd get through this because I am really strong.
>
> *Ashley*

She feels depressed, confused, crazy, anxious, and alone. She wonders how long her conditions of powerlessness and helplessness will persist. She fears the difficulty of her past will forever have the power to simply expand and recapture her. Sometimes she feels there is no escape. Trapped in a struggle with the wounded child within and to break the taboo of silence imposed on her long ago, she feels destined to a life of tremendous difficulty with self-esteem, trust, physical and emotional anguish. She fears she cannot escape from a life forever plagued by some enormous problem. Suicide becomes an attractive option.

> Another suicide attempt took place and they admitted me through emergency. I told the doctor I had abuse issues, my mother was my perpetrator, and I wanted to die. He said, "Oh, what could she do to you? She doesn't have a penis." I said very angrily,

"She's got fingers, she's got a mouth, and she can use objects."
He was quiet after that, but my anger was uncontrollable.

*Ashley*

The mother-daughter incest survivor will describe how lonely and
alone she is. She may believe she is the only one in the world who has
experienced abuse so "out of the ordinary."

Behind my fear is a lot of grief and sorrow for the struggle my
life has always been, and for the isolation and loneliness I can't
seem to escape.

*Louise*

She feels unable to develop a sense of commonality with others in her
social environment and hence perceives herself as markedly different
from others. The isolation imposed on her serves to compound this
belief. Her feeling of aloneness is fed by the family's secretiveness
and society's denial of the existence of the phenomenon of mother-
daughter incest. She may feel so alone that she is unable to tell her
story to anyone. Even in therapy, she may not share her secret, fearful
that the awful truth will drive the trusted person, her therapist, away. She
cannot afford to be left alone once more or to be disbelieved or rejected.

The clinician needs to recognize that the mother-daughter incest
survivor often feels protected by her silence. She may not reveal that
her mother was her abuser. As a child, the secrecy served to keep the
behavior from being uncovered and terminated. She convinced herself that if she tells her secret, her primary relationship to the seemingly omnipotent and often beloved abuser may be threatened (Miller,
1994). The child may be deeply confused by the fact that her mother,
her abuser, is both enemy and lover to her. She may internalize the
abuser to become part of her psychic self. With disclosure, she may risk
losing part of herself. As an adult, in group therapy she may choose to
remain silent for fear of being rejected by group members.

Because I am a mother-daughter incest survivor, I feel so isolated. The group that I was in spoke of the men who abused
them. It took me a long time to say to these women that my
mother abused me. I was afraid the group would reject me.

*Louise*

The helping professional must be open to the possibility that the mother-daughter incest survivor may present with feelings of being trapped all alone in the world. The clinician must attempt to understand and respect the client's position about not being able to control her own life or become a worthwhile person. This message was reinforced time and time again throughout childhood by her mother. The therapist must be cognizant that as a further means of domination and control, the mother-daughter incest victim is often told that surviving in the world is impossible for her without her mother. Essentially she may believe she is possessed and owned by her mother. She may fear that she will not escape her mother's grip and that her mother will never let go. Trapped in fear, self-loathing, and shame, she may believe deep within her core that she will not be anything without her mother. She may enter adolescence and adulthood believing that her existence can only be justified by someone else, which sets her up to fall prey to further victimization, to be used over and over again by someone else.

> I felt I was there for people to use. I would do anything people wanted me to do. I had no idea of wants or needs or anything like that. I remember when I went to university and I had a scholarship. I didn't know what to do with the money. I gave a lot of it away. I didn't know how to spend it. I didn't know how to buy clothes for myself. I'd never bought myself a record or anything like that because I didn't know what I wanted. I didn't know I could have anything I wanted. I didn't have any concept. So much of it was in regards to my mother, so much of my image.
>
> *Michelle*

> I've got the feeling that I don't have the right to say no. My body isn't my own. I don't deserve any better. That this is all men want. This is my total value in life. Not to even be a sexual being for my pleasure but to be a sexual being for their pleasure. That I don't deserve any better.
>
> *Sonia*

For the mother-daughter incest survivor, helplessness and isolation were her core experiences of the trauma. Empowerment and reconnection are the basis of her recovery. In therapy, she will need assistance in the area of self-mastery and self-possession. The therapist will need to encourage her to take concrete steps to increase her sense of power and control, to protect herself from further victimization, and to strengthen her alliance with those she has grown to trust. She will need encouragement to break away from patterns of behavior conditioned by fear, anxiety, self-doubt, self-blame, and guilt. The therapist may encourage the victim to resolve fears concerning survival on her own, and help her learn new ways of thinking and responding in the world. Establishing a degree of control over her bodily and emotional responses reaffirms her sense of power. The therapist can facilitate these changes through encouragement and patience that will enhance the client's self-esteem, self-efficacy, and ability to face her world more confidently.

Counseling may focus on how the mother-daughter incest victim coped with her abuse. The therapist can give the mother-daughter incest survivor respect by honoring her methods of surviving her abuse experience. She can be complimented for her desire to break her silence and break free from her mother's dominance and control. The therapist must acknowledge the mother-daughter incest survivor's inner strength, that despite the extreme physical, sexual, and emotional abuse she experienced throughout her life, she survived. The therapist must acknowledge appreciation of the mother-daughter incest survivor's adaptive resources and how she can utilize her capabilities to enrich her life. The therapist will need to encourage her to feel a sense of pride and healthy admiration of the self, to rejoice in her inner strength, and thus help diminish and compensate her feelings of self-loathing and worthlessness.

The therapist must understand that the mother-daughter incest survivor, similar to other abused children, has difficulty finding alternate attachment figures because the strategies for getting along and surviving in the world tend to alienate her from the very people who might otherwise help her and connect to her. The behavior of many abused children elicits negative reactions from the people around them and repeatedly confirms for the children that they are worthless, incapable of love, and of being loved. It confirms for the mother-daughter incest survivor that she is trapped in a world that treats her as if she is an irritation, and that does not trust her. She believes that she was set up by her mother for a lifetime of abnormal, unsatisfying interpersonal relationships.

Individual or group therapy can speed up the recovery process for the mother-daughter incest survivor and give her experience in building trusting relationships. Group therapy provides a setting of like-minded adult survivors sharing their recovery experiences. The mother-daughter incest survivor in group therapy can break free from her entanglement and enjoy being herself. She can explore her socialized presuppositions that rendered her exploitable in the past. She can identify and overcome external sources of continued social pressure that confine her in a victim role. Experiencing loving relationships and learning to appreciate who and what she is can be healing for the survivor.

In group therapy, she learns to distinguish between feeling autonomous while remaining interconnected to others. She discovers that she can take a position and maintain her own point of view and her own boundaries while valuing those of others. As she creates a new identity, she opens herself to the possibility of new alliances. She is ready to seek mutual friendships and deepen relationships. The deepening of connection and attachment is also apparent within the therapeutic alliance. There is less intensity and more security, more spontaneity and humor. The client has a greater capacity for self-regulation and an increased tolerance for inner conflict. With this renewed appreciation for herself comes a changed appreciation for the therapist. She becomes more forgiving of her own limitations as well as those of her therapist (Herman, 1992).

Farther along in her recovery process, the mother-daughter incest survivor may take the initiative to confront others, to readily reveal her secrets, to challenge societal indifference, and to accuse those who have abused her. By making a public complaint or accusation, she defies the perpetrator's attempts to silence and control her. She may declare to her family that their rule of silence that preserved their secret has been irrevocably broken. In so doing, the mother-daughter incest survivor, without need for confirmation and without fear of consequences, renounces the burden of shame, guilt, and responsibility for the abuse. She is able to place this burden where it properly belongs, with her mother. She draws power from her ability to speak the truth. She is secure in the knowledge that simply her willingness to confront her mother indicates that she has overcome one of the most terrible consequences of her abuse. By speaking about the unspeakable, she feels connected to a power larger than herself, that she is helping others and assisting their recovery process as well as hers.

In summary, the therapist needs to be open to the possibility of mother-daughter incest. Denial of the mother-daughter incest survivor's abuse experience will touch her shame and contribute to her trauma by depriving her of an opportunity in therapy for resolution of her pain, anger, and grief. Therapy may mark the beginning for the client to experience a safe and consistent environment within which to explore the abuse experience, a place where she can go and not feel trapped. Through therapy, the mother-daughter incest survivor can realize that she is a good person, that she needs to, and is capable of, connecting with people in positive, healthy ways so she can affirm her own sense of self-worth. She can empower herself by understanding what happened to her as a child, and making friends with her past. The therapist can empower her by having her take charge of the planning of her sessions. She can become the maker of ground rules rather than the one who automatically obeys them. The therapist can empower her by acknowledging her courage and daring. She is no longer confined by secrecy; she has nothing more to hide. She no longer feels trapped with no place to go or possessed by her traumatic past. She is in possession of herself, and in control of becoming the person she wants to be. In the process of reconciling with herself, she is able to create a new self by drawing on and integrating those aspects of herself that she most values from the time before the abuse, during the abuse itself, and from the recovery process. She becomes more forgiving of herself and as she actively engages in the rebuilding of her life, she becomes more generous and accepting of the memory of the traumatized self, and of her powerlessness to stop the abuse.

# Chapter 5

# Double-Crossed: Betrayal and Grief

I think the most difficult thing is that I always wanted a mom. No matter how bad she was I just really wanted a mom, somebody to hold me, all that kind of stuff. It's such a longing. I have some really good friends that I'm intimate with, but it doesn't fill that void. I have men friends that I'm really intimate with too, and that doesn't fill the void either. It's totally different and a different kind of holding and wanting to be held.

*Beatrice*

Society recognizes child abuse as a breach of faith with the community of humanity. Child abuse is a story of misused power, exploitation, and the betrayal of innocence. Incest is about betrayal of trust. It is usually an offense committed by adults against children, by the powerful against the weak.

According to the literature (Ogilvie and Daniluk, 1995; Miller, 1994), the closer the relationship with the abuser, the deeper the sense of betrayal. Because their mother was their abuser, mother-daughter incest survivors undoubtedly experience an intense sense of betrayal. They experienced betrayal because they were harmed as children by someone they had been vitally dependent upon, by someone who was expected to be their adult protector. They experienced helplessness without support and imposed secrecy. Because of the strength of the mother-daughter dyad, victims of mother-daughter incest, perhaps more so than other incestuous dyads, feel betrayed, deserted, and rejected since their abuser was their mother.

Given cultural definitions of motherhood and societal perceptions of the protective strength of the mother-daughter dyad, the practitioner will need to anticipate that mother-daughter incest survivors will present in therapy with a profound sense of betrayal of trust by their mothers. This theme of profound betrayal may be accentuated more than any other theme by mother-daughter incest survivors. Based on their belief that their mother's common gender should have resulted in deep empathic understanding and care, the sense of betrayal that is also commonly expressed by survivors of other types of sexual abuse, seems to be even more extreme for many mother-daughter incest survivors. Mother-daughter incest survivors may not express hostility or rage toward their fathers for not protecting them. Although they often describe their fathers as being emotionally and physically absent, they reiterate their belief that the mother in the family is responsible for protecting and nurturing her children. They believe that their mothers abdicated their primary role as protector and abandoned their responsibility by placing their own needs above the needs of their daughters.

Mother-daughter incest survivors feel that they received little nurturance, education, and guidance from their mothers when they were growing up. They grieve the fact that gaps appear in their upbringing and that they failed to acquire particular abilities and knowledge, which children who have traditional upbringings take for granted. To mother-daughter incest survivors, life meant surviving the challenges of their abuse experience. They had little energy for anything else. They were cut off from the outside world, discouraged from taking part in extracurricular school activities, and denied peer relationships. Perhaps they coped with their abuse experience in maladaptive ways as a result of their emotional and psychological problems. Their understanding of themselves, others, and the future was distorted by their perpetrators. Their entire personality structure, including cognitive and emotional functioning, was shaped by reprehensible mothers who provided a life of brutality and abomination (Herman, 1992).

> It's really weird because after working years through issues around sexual abuse by males when this came up around my mother perpetrating, I was absolutely devastated. I felt the most profound sense of betrayal, more so than what I felt around the males. It felt far worse, not expected. I felt completely shattered because it was my mother. I always knew that I was neglected and unprotected by her. That she had limits around that. If anyone would ask me why did this memory of your mother come up so late in the process, why did it take so long to emerge, my response was, "Because it's the most devastating—it's my mother,

the one that's supposed to protect me and nurture me." There's such a conflict in terms of that kind of violation. I couldn't go to her to be physically nurtured, held, hugged, or kissed. When I got physically sick, she got mad at me. That was very difficult, so I had to basically bring myself up and take care of myself. And having to look after her and protect her, while not having any emotional intimacy with her. Having to suppress my rage. The emotional abandonment whereby there was a lot of times in my life when I was very traumatized, abused, when most kids would have gone to their mother crying, I couldn't do that. I just had to shut it down.

*Mable*

The mother-daughter incest survivor may express grief and depression over the absence of a trusted figure and that she has been deceived, misled, deserted, or taken in by her mother. She feels tremendous anger that her mother had the right to inflict horrible abuse on her and get away with it. She feels double-crossed and ripped off because she was denied the opportunity to identify with a caregiving mother. She experiences confusion and a profound sense of loss that her mother did not bond with her. Instead, she experienced her mother as deficient and defective in her mothering role. She may feel extreme hostility and anger as a result of being cheated out of a healthy mother-daughter relationship.

I'm left with this legacy. I'm the one who has to live with it. She does whatever she does; she copes her way. She'll die soon and it will be over for her, but it's never going to be over for me. Therapy is not cheap. I have to work hard to be able to go to therapy to just get through life. My whole life is so wrapped up in it. It's stopped me from having things that I really want, what my heart desires, just to have some loving. In my fantasies, I meet this little old woman who wants to adopt me. And she's not my mother's age. She's like a grandmother because that's safe for me. I can deal with that. I have trouble with people being my mother's age. Part of me still wants the woman who raised me to love me. But that part is getting smaller. I felt so much hatred for her. I'm still working with the anger and the rage. It's taken a long time for me to be able to feel it. I just don't want to have anything to do with my mother. Yes there's a part of me, the little child, that would love to have a mother, that still longs for her, but not my mother. I fantasize about the things I would have liked to receive. Like a lot of touching and warmth, being close. Being told that I was wanted. Someone to spend time with me.

*Sonia*

The practitioner will need to be open to the mother-daughter incest survivor's feelings of extreme anger as a result of being deceived and ostracized by a society that denies the existence of mother-daughter incest. The practitioner needs to be aware that the mother-daughter incest survivor is likely to present with strong feelings that she was thrust aside, ridiculed, scorned, and hated throughout her life. As a result of society's disbelief that mother-daughter incest can occur, feelings of betrayal, of being defective, different, and stigmatized for survivors appear to be exacerbated. For these women, feelings of detachment are manifested in an impaired ability to trust and an aversion to intimacy. Mother-daughter incest survivors emphasize that because they feel they cannot trust their own mother, they have an impaired ability to trust themselves and others. They fear intimacy and experience difficulty with interpersonal relationships. They often feel confused about their relationships with other women and particularly struggle with trusting them. They may be unable to connect with their therapist and also experience difficulty with self-mastery and control.

The therapist should note, however, that these women may experience an intense need to regain trust and security. They may long for relationships and connection. The practitioner must pay particular attention to the therapeutic alliance and to the maintenance of healthy boundaries between client and therapist. The helping professional needs to be aware that these women may feel that they will never get what they want, that they are under a permanent cloud of the mother's betrayal. The process of recovery for these women may be long and arduous.

My relationship was chaotic and insane with my mother. I didn't have a relationship with her. She was only in take mode. I could give, give, give, give, and she would only take, take, take, take. I could never make her happy. I remember spending three weeks looking for a Christmas present for her. Right up to the end, I ended up trying to please her and to get her to love me.

*Alana*

Because of their abuse experience, they do not have a positive identity with their mothers. Connectedness is missing, as well as mutual caring that is found in healthy mother-daughter interactions. As children, perhaps they were never held or told they were loved. No tactile, verbal, or spiritual nurturance occurred. Perhaps they were told they were ugly and that their mother was thinking of ways to get rid of them. They often felt like muted nonentities.

> I realize I lost so much of my childhood. There was a lack of nurturing, never any trips with my mom. We didn't go to the library, we never went skating or tobogganing. I did absolutely nothing other than accept abuse from my mother. There were no warm, fuzzy feelings. There were no "I love you's." I don't know whether or not it's a fairy tale. You hear about other people's mothers, how they care about them, call them and have this really casual relationship where they go shopping together or they ask how your workday went. I never had any of that. It's very difficult not having that with your mom. I've waited my whole life to have somebody who cares about me. I feel such a loss—you don't ever get over that. I really envy other people who have that sense of connectedness. I have a hole in my soul that never seems to get filled. You can't go adopting other people's mothers.

*Alana*

As adults, they fear themselves to be incomplete or insufficient as women. They feel double-crossed because they were denied empathic communication and mutual attentiveness with their mothers, which affected their self-esteem and self-affirmation. They continue to lack confidence, strength, and competence in their relational capacities. No mechanism was available for self-validation and self-definition. They still feel imprisoned because the captor has total control over their existence and unlimited access to their bodies. The multiple violation and deprivation they experienced in childhood at

the hands of their mothers has a traumatic and devastating effect on
their lives.

> I really feel badly about the fact that she was the way she was. I
> wanted with all my heart for us to have a better relationship than
> we did, and I could never have that. It didn't matter what I did. It
> wasn't attainable. The way that it's manifested itself in my adult
> life is that I've quite often been with men who are also unavail-
> able emotionally. When you are not able to resolve the child-
> hood issues, you are unfortunately enslaved by them until you
> can recognize a pattern and begin to make conscious decisions
> not to fall into the pattern.

*Alana*

Throughout childhood, adolescence, and adulthood, they are given
the overwhelming message from the world that their experience of
abuse was not real. It could not have occurred; therefore it was invented, made up, and something the survivor was doing to herself.

> Nobody helped me. I told my friend's mother about my mother
> abusing me, and she told me what a terrible kid I was.

*Christine*

As a result, the survivor is forced to self-blame for something that
was done to her. When she expresses grief, pain, anger, or fear, the response she often receives is "How could you make up such a story?
There must be something wrong with you." So she is forced to doubt
herself, to mistrust her perceptions. Because the truth of her experience is so difficult for the mother-daughter incest survivor to face, she
will often vacillate in reconstructing her story. Denial of reality
makes her feel crazy, and acceptance of the full reality seems light
years beyond what any human being can bear.
    From a place of bewilderment, she often asks the unfathomable
question: "Why?" She also confronts another equally incomprehen-
sible question: "Why me?" She believes the answers to these questions are beyond human understanding. In order to develop a full understanding of her traumatic past, she must examine the moral questions

of guilt and accountability and restore a system of belief that makes sense of her undeserved suffering (Dalenberg, 2000). She faces the daunting task of reconstructing her own shattered assumptions about meaning, order, and justice in the world.

In therapy, she will attempt to find the wholeness that was stolen from her in childhood. She will endeavor to overcome a personality structure within which she tells herself that she is not valuable and not wanted. Even though her voice may have grown stronger throughout the years, she still gets frustrated, grieves, and feels deeply betrayed by a world that believes she is telling an impossible lie, that mothers do not sexually abuse children and that the mother is the victim. Familial denial, professional denial, and societal denial effectively prevent her from getting treatment.

> When I told my friend about my mother's abuse of me, it was interesting because what I heard was like "That isn't so bad. That isn't as bad as your father; she was probably just lonely." They excused her. I had a lot of trouble for a long time with what I call feministic or people who are so against men as being abusive. In their minds, women can't do anything wrong.

> *Michelle*

The mother-daughter incest survivor in therapy is likely to describe a lifetime of severe loss which has disrupted her pattern of attachments and how she constructs meaning in her life. These losses induce tremendous grief because the survivor's ability to experience life as meaningful is disrupted.

> I've never had somebody to hang in there with me. That's been a pattern. I've always attracted women who were not very good friends, who didn't see me as a person. It's such a big loss. It feels like I've been in a depressed state and that things are breaking down, that I'm breaking down. Having to surrender is to realize that I'm only human. I've lost most of my friends through the past three years. Most people can't deal with it. I feel like I'm the only one, that I'm the oddball, that I'm different and damaged.

> *Sonia*

As the mother-daughter incest survivor faces the task of grieving what was lost, she also mourns what was never hers to lose. She grieves the irreplaceable childhood that was stolen from her. She mourns the loss of foundation of basic trust, and the belief in a good parent. As she comes to a place of recognition that she was not responsible for her fate, she is able to confront the existential despair that she could not face in childhood. Without the inner image of a caring mother, she doubts that she can survive in her world. This puts her at high risk for suicide. Her suicidality may arise from a calm, flat rational decision to reject a world where such atrocities occur. She may feel that she is already among the dead because her capacity for love has been destroyed.

The therapist will need to understand that descent into mourning is the most necessary and most dreaded task in the recovery process for many survivors (Baures, 1994). Mother-daughter incest survivors frequently describe the task as insurmountable. They often dwell on the fact that if they allow themselves to grieve, it will never stop. Some survivors may resist mourning traumatic loss out of fear and shame. Some refuse to address their grief as a way of denying victory to their abusive mothers.

As the mother-daughter incest survivor explores the most unbearable moments of her trauma, she may be rendered speechless. The therapist will need to encourage her to communicate nonverbally: to draw, paint, or sculpt, or to write down her story. The therapist may need to remind the client that their mutual goal is to bring the story into the room where it can be spoken and heard. Following the basic principle of empowerment during the remembering and mourning stage, the therapist is witness and ally in whose presence the mother-daughter incest survivor can speak the unspeakable. He or she will need to be cognizant of the fact that avoiding traumatic memories leads to stagnation in the recovery process; approaching them too precipitately leads to fruitless and damaging reliving of the trauma. Decisions regarding pacing and timing will need meticulous attention and frequent review by the client and therapist in concert. The course of therapy may need to slow down if active exploration of the trauma becomes too much for the client to handle (Pearlman and Saakvitne, 1995).

The process of therapy can enable the mother-daughter incest survivor to express her feelings of grief, anger, fear, sadness, denial, and shock for her losses. It allows her to take full control of her recovery by taking responsibility for it. Grieving will allow for more and more healing and acceptance. The process of recovery from grief for the mother-daughter incest survivor will involve reconstructing meaning by rebuilding the continuity of life, making sense of what happened and assimilating it to present circumstances in a purposeful manner. She can learn what she missed in her past and strive to put it back into her life. She can put aside her negative beliefs and replace them with positive ones. She can become empowered by learning to love and cherish the innocent child that she was. She can empower herself by allowing herself to not be a victim of further abuse.

The therapist must reframe the client's mourning as an act of courage and an important part of her healing. Through mourning everything that was taken from her, she can discover her strengths and resilience. During the mourning process, the mother-daughter incest survivor must come to terms with her desire for revenge. Repetitive revenge fantasies, which often arise from her experience of complete helplessness, often reverse the roles of victim and perpetrator, allow her to retaliate, provide her the opportunity to alleviate the terror, shame, and pain of her experience, and restore her own sense of power. These fantasies may also be extremely frustrating, exacerbate the victim's feelings of horror, and degrade her self-image. In the process of remembering and mourning, where she comes to terms with the impossibility of getting even and vents her rage in safety, her helpless fury gradually transforms into a more powerful and satisfying form of anger, righteous indignation (Herman, 1992). This transformation allows her to free herself from feeling that she is a monster, imprisoned in revenge fantasies. She regains a sense of power without becoming a criminal.

The major work of remembering and mourning is accomplished when she reclaims her own history, renews hope and energy for engagement with life, and pursues her aspirations for the future. Establishing new relationships enables her to shed her evil, stigmatized identity. Through new relationships, she recognizes that she no longer has anything to hide. She develops a new self, and reclaims her world. As she builds a new life within a radically different culture from the one she left behind, and emerges from an atmosphere of total control, she simultaneously feels the wonder and uncertainty of freedom. She often feels like a visitor to a foreign country. She will come to a place where she recognizes that her traumatic experience no longer is central to her life. She has mourned the old self destroyed by the abuse. She has challenged old beliefs that once dominated and gave meaning to her existence. She may reach a renewal stage, the spring after the winter, where she feels creative, energized, and empowered from her grief process. Over time, she may come to consider how and why her mother behaved as she did. She may gain understanding of how things developed, which may allow her to move to a place of forgiveness and reconciliation.

> It was only toward the end of her life that I came to reconcile with her and to the realization that I really liked this woman. Before therapy, I had realized that my mother was in a lot of pain for most of her life. When she finished her change of life, it was like a role reversal for her. This very violent woman, I saw her change.

*Iris*

> Silent tears, screaming,
> Pain, a beast's hate and love.
> Her hands create Tortured Tears,
> Our tears create children to survive.
> Our hands hold strong
> Her Hands no more.
> Tortured tears,
> No more silenced,
> All have a voice.

*Gloria and The Chorus Line*

# Chapter 6

# Identification with and Differentiation from Mother

Everything I did was done out of the sense that I don't want to be like her, I don't want to be her. It was like this big revelation to me. I was being like her in trying to be opposite to her. I was still really tied to her, so much in my energy, being determined to be different than her rather than being who I was. I guess I wanted to be everything that my mother wasn't. I think one of my biggest fears through my teens and early twenties was that I'd end up in a mental institution and never get out.

*Michelle*

The mother-daughter incest survivor may report that she struggles with identifying with and differentiating from her mother. She struggles with distancing herself from her mother and developing a healthy sense of personal identity. She cannot connect and define herself in terms of her own identity as a woman. She may feel a tremendous sense of guilt about strong feelings of loyalty toward her mother, or lack thereof. She may feel guilty about saying anything negative about her mother or trying to live life differently and separately from her.

I felt sorry for her. I still remember once as late as grade twelve, I did it all my life. I would hurry home from school to see if she was still alive at the same time wishing she wouldn't be. That was really confusing for me. Part of me wanted to nurture her, yet part of me hoped she would die. I know my whole goal was to save my mother. I had such a strong need to save her or change her. When I was around her I couldn't stand her touching me. I would feel really guilty if I didn't or couldn't be nice to her. I would try to be nice. It was really phony.

*Michelle*

The mother-daughter incest survivor has not had the opportunity to learn boundaries. She may have no idea in terms of where she ends psychologically and physically and where another person begins. She may not recognize that she is entitled to be a separate self, a distinct identity. She may not be able to conceptualize that she has her own needs, desires, and feelings. Since boundaries have not been modeled or defined for her, she may not be able to set limits. Incest has obliterated all of this.

> I just felt like I wasn't a separate person. I was part of her. I was responsible for her being happy or being unhappy. The closer I tried to get to her the more she would push me away. When I would back up or withdraw, she would come closer and drag me back. This kind of push/pull type of thing, a sticky, gooey dance. I still have to work really hard to overcome negative thoughts, negative thinking. I hear her voice in that negativity. It sounds exactly like her. She's very much alive in me. I don't like the feeling of being depressed because that reminds me of her. I guess I see her when I feel like I'm a victim, when I'm manipulative. As I'm healing, I see my patterns and how I sometimes behave like her.

*Sonia*

Many mother-daughter incest survivors find it difficult to think of their mothers as being all bad. They may describe her as brutal and incredibly cruel, yet caring and compassionate. In attempts to make sense of the abuse experience, mother-daughter incest survivors find it difficult to believe that their mother could do anything wrong because she was supposed to take care of her children. They may have happy memories of good times and helpful lessons that their mothers taught them. These pleasant memories may feed confusion and distort reality for the survivor.

The mother-daughter incest survivor may remember her mother as being beautiful and witty, as having a great sense of humor. Perhaps she was the envy of many of the neighbors. Perhaps many of the children in the neighborhood shared with the daughter that they wished her mother was their mother. Maybe she was successful in her profession, respected by many for her business endeavors and her community involvement. The daughter, however, will also remember the physical brutality, the sexual intrusiveness, the ongoing powerful words that annihilated the good feelings she had about herself, leaving a devastating impact on her life.

> She could be loving at times. There were periods when she would be fun, but then she'd fabricate something which would ruin it all. She would accuse me of doing something or not doing something which would make me leave and withdraw. She'd flip right out.
>
> *Ashley*

The therapist will need to be sensitive to this confusion that the daughter has in terms of who her mother is and how the daughter experienced her. The therapist must be cognizant of the profound consequences of the daughter's witness of her mother's impaired psychological and emotional functioning, and the absence and distortion when abuse occurs of the support, distance, and modeling that are central to all parent-child relationships.

> I don't want to be similar to her in any respect. I don't want to look at anything the same way that she does because to me that would be too close that I might carry her mental illness. That's a really big fear that somehow I'll be crazy like her.
>
> *Taylore*

The daughter may feel that she is mentally ill and needs to be institutionalized or incarcerated. She may blame herself and experience feelings that she is the perpetrator; she may hate herself and experience tremendous rage that she may be unable to direct toward her mother. People may believe that she is soft-spoken, self-confident, and self-assured. At her very core, however, she may feel totally incomplete and insufficient. She may be a superb mother, but deep inside herself she fears that she is inadequate in her maternal role, just as her mother was. She fears that she has the capacity to be like her mother, the perpetrator, yet awareness of this issue helps her to recognize the difference. She is still unable, however, to trust herself, especially with children, for fear she may perpetrate against them.

Given the fact that mother-daughter incest survivors have experienced unhealthy role modeling, the clinician must be open to the possibility that mother-daughter incest survivors, who are mothers themselves, may present with deep concern and fear about continuing the cycle of abuse. They undoubtedly will feel anxious and afraid of victimizing their own children or even someone else's. The therapist must be able to ask the survivor if she has offended against another due to the fact that she may be playing out her own sexual abuse as a child.

Therapy will focus on the struggles the mother-daughter incest survivor experiences with separation and identity issues. The practitioner must be open to the mother-daughter incest survivor's seemingly contradictory position in terms of identifying with and differentiating from her mother.

> I remember having very mixed emotions toward her. Here was a part of me that loved her as a child and wanted so desperately to be loved and accepted by her. When I was growing up, I kept saying, "I will never be like you, the bitch from hell." There was a lot of hate and animosity toward her when I was growing up. A lot of mixed feelings—I loved her, but I didn't like her. I hated her, despised her. There was such confusion. If anyone hurt my mother or said anything against her, I defended her like a knight in shining armor.
>
> *Iris*

The therapeutic process may provide a safe place for the mother-daughter incest survivor to express feelings of extreme anxiety and fear of being like her mother. The practitioner will need to understand that in her desire to be different from her mother, she may change her physical appearance and deny her femininity.

> If you know you are different from her, then you are free. She's gone and you can let it go. Every day, every single day, I back into it, into the fear that I will be like her.
>
> *Patti*

I look like her, and that was one of the reasons besides the abuse that I wanted to kill myself. I would go out of my way to be unlike her. Anything I would do or say that was like her I would be alerted by my siblings so I would go out of my way to be unlike her.

*Ashley*

Some survivors of mother-daughter incest may react to their impaired identification with their mother by not wanting to have children, or avoiding a maternal role.

When I was a teen and even a young adult, I wasn't going to have children at all. I was scared because I had been told all my life that I was so much like my mother. If I were to have children I would be just like her.

*Louise*

It may be important for the helping professional to acknowledge to the survivor that the process of separation and identity formation may trigger feelings of low self-esteem, helplessness, powerlessness, fearfulness, and depression, which manifest in poor interpersonal relationships. During therapy, this difficulty with differentiation, interdependence, and the establishment of physical and psychological boundaries for the client can be identified in order for her to be consciously aware of her difficulty with identity formation. The survivor will need to develop her own individuality separate from her mother and other significant people in her life, to define and regulate herself so she can determine who she is.

I just felt like I was falling apart the whole time. My whole struggle was to keep out of the insane asylum. That was my goal. It was like a fog. It was like I was trying to make a life separate from that, not realizing that you can't. I was living my husband's life rather than my own. I followed his dreams because I had none of my own. I didn't have anything I wanted for myself other than not to be crazy.

*Michelle*

I've done everything in my power to not be like her. That's what freaked me out. I'd get to forty and end up like her. Somebody would come along and compare me to her and I'd just go nuts because I've worked hard at trying to be different. I just want to develop some sort of my own identity. Even though she wants me to be a certain way, I've gone in the opposite direction.

*Jacqueline*

The practitioner will need to be cognizant that, as she struggles to differentiate and distance herself from her mother, at the same time she may need to connect with her mother in defining her own identity as a woman and as a mother. She may be reluctant to disown her mother because that may mean rejecting part of her own identity or denying who she is. She may describe difficulty in identity formation because of her enmeshment with her mother.

It's hard for me too because I don't want to reject everything of my mother in me. A person can't be a whole person if you're trying to deny half of what you are.

*Beth*

The critical developmental issues in working with adult female survivors of maternal incestuous abuse include identification, differentiation, interdependence, and the establishment of physical and psychological boundaries. Mother-daughter incest survivors experience difficulties in the development of a healthy sense of personal identity. They will need assistance and support in working through fears of being like their mothers. In particular, they will need help in seeing themselves as different from the women who abused them. Eventually they may find some kernel of value, some positive experience that was not abusive. Once the pain lessens, they may expand their perspective about their mother. Once they get past their anger and begin to access their hurt and loss, they may begin the process of identifying and integrating into their own identity the healthier, nonabusive parts of their mother's personality that were apparent when the mother was not being abusive.

I did a ritual at my parents' graves. I told them that I loved them and that I forgave them. I was through being angry. I have no anger left. The memories are there. I can't rewrite the memories. I can actually say I love them. I want them to find peace. I really want my mom to find peace. I want her to be made whole and to feel love because she never really felt love. I want her to know that I really do appreciate who she was as a person. Some of the things other people saw in her, I see in her now. I don't bear her any animosity. I love and appreciate what she was trying to do. Because she didn't have an education she didn't know a lot of stuff. She felt cheated. I felt cheated. I can now associate that part of empathy toward her.

*Iris*

# Chapter 7

# Impaired Sexual Development

I am working and struggling toward understanding my sexuality and I want to say maybe it's no thanks to my mum. Sexual feelings are slowly coming forth, and I'm listening to them but I'm in a state of confusion. I shut down and have no feelings, and so the sexual tension rises. I have such fear around being intimate with people. I take it very slowly around women, and I know it's connected to the abuse, all these issues around intimacy and trust and sexuality.

*Lisa*

Mother-daughter incest survivors, similar to survivors of other forms of abuse, may display various symptoms of impaired sexual development throughout their lives. They are likely to experience conflicts in intimacy and trust. In particular, they may feel confused about behavior in intimate relationships. As children, they were probably confused about the function of sex in affectionate relationships. They may struggle with blending emotional intimacy and sexual activity. Perhaps they developed an aversion to all sexual experiences and to intimacy.

Unsureness about what love is has been an issue that I've lived all my life. It goes back to when I was growing up. I didn't know what love was. Love was a mother flying off at the handle, beating me black and blue, and being abusive, sexually abusive as well. I realized part of it was my dad, who loved me and cared and protected me, was physically abusive to me as well.

*Iris*

A mother-daughter incest survivor often experiences herself as being easy prey for further victimization primarily due to feelings of powerlessness and shame. When her sexual boundaries were violated by her mother, she learned that she did not have rights. As an adult, the pattern is set for the survivor to feel powerless to say no, to resist. For adult survivors of mother-daughter incest, feeling in charge of their bodies and their sexuality is a huge battle that they fight their entire lives. Setting physical and psychological boundaries is difficult for them. Establishing and maintaining rules for being sexual becomes a real challenge. They have limited understanding of how to feel in charge of choosing to be physical or sexual. They have been held back by rules and attitudes and negative messages about themselves and their sexuality. To them, living life to its fullest and enjoying their sexuality is inconceivable.

Mother-daughter incest survivors experience difficulty with sexual identity; at times they may be promiscuous; sometimes they may avoid and fear sex; other times they may be sexually dysfunctional or demonstrate repetitive sexual behavior during late childhood and early adolescence. Sexual contact in a child's memory may be associated with revulsion, fear, anger, a sense of powerlessness, or other negative emotions, and these feelings may become generalized as an aversion to all sexual experiences in intimacy. Traumatic sexuality causes confusion about the role of sex in affectionate relationships. If child victims have traded sex for affection, they may perceive this as the normal way to give and receive affection.

Victims of interfamilial sexual abuse generally have not had appropriate models on which to base their understanding of intimacy or sexuality. They may have witnessed constant fighting and/or complete distance between parents. Often the only attention and affection they received stemmed from the sexual relationship with the abuser (Tower, 1988). Some may commit themselves to a lifestyle of celibacy because they fear they would become paralyzed by flashbacks during sex. Many choose to be celibate because of their history of numerous sexually and emotionally abusive relationships. Some mother-daughter incest survivors experience confusion about their sexual orientation.

It's like not being able to differentiate between myself and her—not being able to—I don't think that separation took place, even though yeah, it's like the connection was a sexual one and then there was no separation. I would at certain times adopt certain behaviors, sexual behaviors of my mother in my life. I would be asexual for a while, and then I'd be sexual and feel really like a whore. I think that's what my mother was like too. Trying to explore issues of possible bisexuality. I know that not always, but sometimes, sexual abuse can confuse your sexual orientation. I feel like it closed a door to something that maybe would have been there naturally.

*Mable*

I went through a period of time when I was confused about my sexual orientation. My surrogate mom was so close to me and I checked it out if she ever wanted to have sex with me because to me love meant sex. Loving another woman meant sex. I wanted to know if she had any inclination that way. Of course, she said no and that we had a healthy relationship, and that she wouldn't cross those boundaries. So I felt safe and secure and that I could trust her. I learned how I could have an appropriate relationship with a mother-figure.

*Ashley*

Tower (1988) posits that it is not uncommon for a mother-daughter incest survivor to choose lesbian partners in later life. The survivor is searching for a nonexploitive mother figure to love her for herself and not for her sexual acquiescence. Survivors who are not lesbian may be plagued by fears and confusion about the meaning of their feelings toward other women.

I think that I was in the victim role for a long time with all those people sexually assaulting me. I thought there was something really wrong with me. I even questioned my own identity as a woman. I thought, wait a second, am I gay? I could relate to my son's feelings around being gay because a man sexually assaulted him. Of course not, but you still question yourself, and ask what is wrong with yourself. For a while I was totally confused. Did I want a man or a woman? I didn't know what it was. I didn't know who I was sexually.

*Iris*

The helping professional must understand that in response to feelings of worthlessness and powerlessness, many sexual abuse victims fall prey to further victimization. The message that mother-daughter incest survivors received throughout their childhood and adolescence was that mastering their own lives or becoming a worthwhile person was impossible. The only way they could justify their existence was to be used over and over by someone else. These women repeatedly find themselves in extremely vulnerable positions due to feeling unworthy of respect and thus deserving further victimization.

As children and adolescents, they may engage in sexual preoccupations and repetitive sexual behavior such as masturbation or compulsive sex play. During adolescence and beyond, perhaps as an attempt to gain some control over their bodies and their sexuality, they may alternate between being promiscuous or being socially and sexually withdrawn. Some children who have been victimized become sexually aggressive and victimize peers or younger children. Victimized girls may wonder whether their sexual desirability has been impaired and whether later sexual partners will discover this (Finkelhor and Browne, 1985). In response to feeling that they have little control in their lives, they may experience an excessive need to dominate others or take control over situations, especially sexual situations.

> I always took the initiative with sex as a teenager. I had to have control over the first time we had sex.
>
> *Taylore*

> I would fake a seizure whenever I was pressed into sex or beaten, and it worked.
>
> *Christine*

The therapist needs to be open to the possibility that some women may use alcohol or drugs to mask difficulties with their sexuality. They may experience such sexual conflicts as not wanting to be touched, inability to achieve orgasm, or finding intercourse physically painful. These problems are often related to trauma brought on by the abuse. The memory of what took place may be too painful, and it may create too much conflict for these women to enjoy adult sexual experiences.

I was damaged by the abuse by men definitely, but it's like damage done by her to my sexuality affects me in relationships with men because I feel like I don't deserve them. The sense of hopelessness sets in that I'll never have a successful relationship with a man. Whatever you want to call successful, one that works. Or even have one period or be deserving of any kind of nice male love and affection. I remember once having this orgasm all by myself, and I had a flash of it's the first time I ever really had that, even though I've enjoyed sex for a long time with men. A flash of a window where my mother was, like my God, she's not in my body right now. I really feel like a woman, and she's not in my body and I feel sexual and I feel really liberated. It was amazing. It lasted about a minute or two, and then it all came back. It's almost like having this ghost come back into my body and there it is. It's still there. It's like she had left for two minutes, and I really think that comes from the sexual abuse by her.

*Mable*

The helping professional will need to be aware that those victims who become promiscuous may be doing so because of a compulsive, self-destructive expression of conflict. Through repeated sexual contact, victims may be trying to work through their anxiety regarding experiences of sexual abuse. At the same time, they may be attempting to fill themselves up with as much human attention as they can acquire, even if it is of a sexual nature.

The therapist needs to encourage the survivor to accept her body and her sexuality. The mother-daughter incest survivor will need to be encouraged to reclaim her body and her sexuality and to experience sex as a choice rather than as an infliction imposed on her. She needs to set her own boundaries and rules for being sexual. The therapist can remind the survivor that she has the right to get to know herself sexually and to express her sexual wants and desires. She will need to pay attention to her emotional needs, to when she wants affection and when she does not.

The therapist will need to normalize for the mother-daughter incest survivor that sexual intimacy presents a particular barrier for survivors of sexual trauma. The therapist may draw from trauma theory that addresses posttraumatic sexual dysfunction and the therapeutic goal of enhancing the survivor's control over every aspect of her sexual life. The therapist should encourage the mother-daughter incest survivor to take charge of her sexuality, to choose when to be physical or sexual, to say no when she wants to, to share herself with someone she trusts, and to acknowledge what stimulates her and what turns her off. The mother-daughter incest survivor will need to define for herself and her partner activities that trigger her traumatic memories as well as those that do not.

The survivor needs to understand that she can make healthy choices about a partner, and that an emotionally and sexually fulfilling relationship is possible for her. She can be encouraged to know her partner well enough so that she may share her abuse experience and any problems concerning triggers or recurring dreams. She will need to give herself permission to stop the lovemaking session if she becomes frightened or triggered and to take a break from sex when she needs to. This will become essential in her recovery and key in taking control of her sexuality. She will need to progress slowly toward establishing a trusting relationship with her partner and making decisions regarding disclosure of her abuse experience. Trusting others will definitely be a key issue throughout her lifetime. In time, she will develop her own sense of trust. Even when she trusts, she will still need to be cognizant of what to disclose, to whom, and when.

The mother-daughter incest survivor may feel acute shame because of the uniqueness of her abuse experience. She may feel shame and confusion about responding sexually and enjoying the physical sensations at the hands of her mother. She will need to understand and accept that it is normal for her body to respond sexually to touching. She can be encouraged to forgive herself and show compassion and understanding if she was promiscuous as an adolescent or young adult. She needs to be complimented for changing old patterns of sexual behavior that put her at risk. It is vital that the therapist accept that she will battle the two taboos, of incest and homosexuality. She may even question her sexual orientation and feel confused and alienated about the issue.

Finally, the mother-daughter incest survivor can be encouraged in therapy to examine her underlying beliefs about being female and to restructure rules and attitudes about life and sexuality. She can reflect upon attitudes and where she acquired or learned them. Through the help of a therapist, she can reconstruct rules and attitudes that were forced upon her, in particular those that prevent her from enjoying her life and her sexuality.

> Sex was like do what you want to me, it doesn't matter. If people even mentioned the word "sex" it just triggered so much. I would be so upset. As long as I didn't think about it or relate to it, it didn't have to be there. That's how I felt about my body. The last five years I've done a lot of work around that and changing those attitudes. In terms of my sexuality, I still have a lot of problems in that there's so much poison there. It's just such a huge issue. In regards to my sexuality, it just feels so muddled still. I read that it's supposed to be one of the last areas of healing from that kind of abuse. I guess it does make lots of sense.

> *Michelle*

Negative messages about her sexuality that she learned in childhood and adolescence can be replaced with positive affirmations. The therapist can acknowledge that exploring sexuality is fun. He or she can emphasize that the female body, including genitals, is beautifully designed, that the survivor is lovable, and that it is wonderful to be a woman. The therapist will need to assist the survivor to accept that she is lovable, that her sexual needs are normal, and that she has the right to ask for what she desires sexually. She needs to know that she can receive cuddling and not be sexual, that sexual fantasies and feelings are normal and she can act on these feelings if she chooses to. The therapist needs to emphasize to the mother-daughter incest survivor that she has the physical and emotional strength, the expertise, and the right to care for herself and take charge of her life and her sexuality.

# Chapter 8

# Difficulty Coping

I've tried alcohol, and I've tried cutting myself. I remember when I was little, a time when I thought that if my hands were cut off I would bleed to death and that would be the end. I remember putting my hands in the door of a car, but it didn't work. I just dented them. I couldn't swim, but I remember going to a lake and just running right for the water. I remember another time with my babysitter when I was swinging on a swing. I knew that if I let go that my chances of dying would be pretty high, so I let go. I fell on my head, and I remember a lot of blood. There were so many accidents of my doing. I didn't care, and I just wanted to die.

*Penny*

Mother-daughter incest survivors often exhibit self-destructive, nonadaptive methods of coping with their sexual victimization at the hands of their mothers. Similar to victims of other forms of sexual abuse, mother-daughter incest survivors demonstrate such behaviors as self-mutilation, suicidal tendencies, substance misuse, depression, promiscuity, eating disorders, suppression or denial of feelings, difficulty with self-mastery and control, as well as physical difficulties and somatic complaints. They feel that they have no control over their lives. A relationship exists between the women's feelings that they have little control over their lives and their excessive need at times to dominate or take control over situations, especially sexual situations, in their lives. Their lives are profoundly impacted by the enormous shame they feel as a result of their abuse experience.

I was always self-destructing. It was like, oh God, I can't have this success, better self-destruct. The minute I attain any success in my life, I tell myself I can't have it now so I guess I'll self-destruct.

*Iris*

From the viewpoint of developmental psychology, people develop basic assumptions about themselves and the world during their early childhood. Children learn basic trust (Erikson, 1970), secure bonding (Bowlby, 1988) and fundamental assumptions (Janoff-Bulman, 1992) that the world is meaningful and kind, and that the individual is worthy. These unconscious beliefs become embedded in the daily experiences of children. They learn specific psychological knowledge about important people in their lives. They learn to influence others and regulate their own emotions.

Abused children also develop basic assumptions and patterns of action that help them cope in the world. Their assumptions about their world and the people in it differ, however, from those of well-cared-for children. For the mother-daughter incest survivor, learning to cope with strong negative emotions and with danger took place in isolation, without support from caretakers. She concludes that she is bad and unworthy, and the world is unjust. She believes that adults are undependable, unpredictable, and untrustworthy.

The mother-daughter incest survivor is denied the opportunity to develop theories and patterns of action with the help of loving adults. She is not allowed the "co-construction of meaning" (Bennett, 1993), nor does she experience sensitivity from the caretaker to her signals as a child. She cannot negotiate the meaning of emotions and learn culturally accepted forms of expression through her relationship with her parents. The mother-daughter incest survivor has not developed an ability to adapt playfully and flexibly to new social situations, and to be present in different social situations through her own input. She is forced to view her world differently. Reality for her involves acting on life-threatening situations, while experiencing herself as nonexistent in a world where nobody cares. Based on survival, her inner logic, her thoughts, and her actions may be more rigid, inflexible, or more vague compared to children who have not been abused. As if danger signals were etched in her memory, she makes decisions and takes action automatically from her logic that tells her the world is not benevolent, violence is inescapable, and people are dangerous.

> I never thought I'd get through it and I didn't want anymore pain or sorrow. I just wanted some peace and quiet and solitude to my life. I felt so bad, like a total failure as a human being, as a mother. I felt that I was the lowest form of life and I didn't want to live and I did not want my kids to go through that with me. I remember driving home one night and there were two semis coming down the highway. My kids were asleep in the back. I wanted to drive out in front of the first semi because I thought if it doesn't kill me and the kids, the second one sure would finish the job. It was the hand of God that came down on my hands until both semis went past. That was such a struggle for me because I wanted my children to live and at the same time I wanted to die. I would think, *Who would be here to take care of them?* Then I would think, *I'll just take it all, just take it all.*
>
> *Iris*

This logic has been cultivated from a young age, from a childhood that saw her body violated, raped, whipped, and beaten, her ambitions squashed, her intelligence mocked, and her love of family, children, and friends thwarted. Incest has taught her guardedness. As a child she learned not to make choices, not to reason, and not to assess and understand. She learned how to survive in a war zone, a battlefield where she was powerless and helpless (Miller, 1994).

The mother-daughter incest survivor's sense of self is seriously impaired by chronic abuse and neglect. She learns to avoid needing what she cannot get from her parents. She develops a false self that obscures her real needs, desires, and experiences, even from herself. Although restrictive, this adaptive self allowed the mother-daughter incest victim to withstand disappointments and violations. Although this false self allowed the child, and even the adult, to function, it seriously compromises her capacity for attachment.

For the mother-daughter incest survivor, repression, often associated with trauma, may be a protective mechanism. She, like other traumatized individuals, may bury some part of the trauma in the unconscious mind because it is too painful or frightening to keep in consciousness. Her experience of being silenced, having reality distorted, and having to repress her traumatic victimization, may contribute to the development of a false sense of self, which along with the practice of silence and deception, becomes the wellspring for the secrets of adult life.

From a need to mentally escape from the intolerable violence over which they had no control as children, many mother-daughter incest survivors lock into a fantasy world to block out pain, and to help with the chronic grief and loss of a life they thought they were going to have. Daydreaming of a better life is commonplace for mother-daughter incest survivors; it helps them to focus away from the pain they have inside, and to disconnect from feelings. It also allows them to experience play and fantasy as well. The mother-daughter incest survivor often resorts to a wide array of psychological defenses which either wall off the abuse from consciousness or minimize, rationalize, excuse, or deny the abuse. Unable to escape or alter the unbearable reality, the child alters it in her mind. A mother-daughter incest survivor may develop to a fine art the capacity for induced trance or dissociative states. She may develop a kind of "dissociative virtuosity where she learns to ignore severe pain, hide memories in complex amnesias, alter her sense of time, place, or person and induce hallucinations. Sometimes these alterations are deliberate, but often they become automatic, alien, and involuntary" (Herman, 1992, p. 102).

As the survivor struggles with the tasks of adult life, the legacy of her childhood may become increasingly burdensome. Often in the third or fourth decade of her life, the defensive structure, which up to this time profoundly protected the mother-daughter incest survivor, may begin to crumble. The precipitant is often a change in the equilibrium of a close relationship: a marriage breakup, the illness or death of a parent, etc. Often for the mother-daughter incest survivor, it is the birth of a child, especially a female child, which precipitates the crisis. She can hold the facade no longer, and the underlying fragmentation becomes manifest and a breakdown may occur. The collapse can take symptomatic forms that mimic every category of psychiatric disorder. The mother-daughter incest survivor often fears that she is going insane or that she will have to die.

Many adult survivors of maternal sexual abuse become obsessed about exercise because it helps them to get rid of feelings, to burn them off and sweat them away. They may develop eating disorders (anorexia, bulimia, overeating) as they hide out from their feelings and the world.

> When I got to be thirteen, I was a chubby kid. Since age ten, my mother had said to me, "You'll have to grow up, be really smart, or you'll have to marry somebody rich because you're going to need plastic surgery because your nose is too big. You're going to be fat and no one is going to want you." I started to starve myself and I went through the anorexia thing. I ended up in the hospital at sixty-two pounds. When I went home after two weeks in the hospital, I got the hell beaten out of me. My mother said to me "What's wrong with you, stupid? Starving yourself, and for what?" I have a lot of problems. Some days, I'll feel really good about myself, but many times I have bad days where I feel depressed. I'll think, *Why did my life have to be like this? Why couldn't I be in a normal family where Mom and Dad go to work, come home, and play games with the kids, where I would grow up and go to college, have a good job, and make a good living?*
>
> *Jacqueline*

For many mother-daughter incest survivors, food may become a focus, a means of control, and a way not to be sexual. To the anorexic, staying thin and wearing baggy clothes hides her womanliness, her sexuality, her body. Refusal to eat may be an active release of anger that allows the anorexic to feel at peace, and comfortable with her body. It may help her to take the stance that no one is going to take charge of her body as had been done to her in childhood. She may want to send the message that nobody is home, that a vault is built around her feelings. To the overeater, food is a comfort, a means of escape, a disconnection from the pain, a way to fill that huge hole in the soul. Her world consists of fear, shame, and hopelessness. When binging, food is the anesthetic. It removes her from the situation.

The mother-daughter incest survivor may become frustrated, horrified, overwhelmed, and depressed by memories during the process of therapy, and begin to engage in self-distancing or self-injurious behaviors. To keep others at a distance and from getting close, the mother-daughter incest survivor may turn to drugs and alcohol.

In high school, I was very disturbed. We'd skip school and get drunk for days, smoke pot and be promiscuous. I just couldn't be alone. Males didn't threaten me at all. I attempted suicide at age sixteen. I overdosed on 222s [prescription painkillers]. That didn't work so I tried to smother myself. After I got out of the hospital, I continued to drink a lot. I was having delirium tremors. I was told I'd die in six months if I didn't quit the booze and drugs. I kept up the lifestyle, but in June of my eighteenth year I had a pregnancy scare and I went down the tubes. I got on my hands and knees at that point and prayed.

*Ashley*

She may engage in other self-injurious behaviors to maintain these boundaries. Self-mutilation, although a painful repetition of childhood trauma, may become a comforting ritual for the mother-daughter incest survivor, a form of taking control of her body. By self-mutilating, she is doing what she wishes and chooses to do with her body. No one can stop her. By self-mutilating, she remains in control, active in her choices, and energetic in her experience of taking charge of her body. Self-injurious behavior may soothe the mother-daughter incest survivor, and protect her from dangerous closeness to others. It may awaken her from her numbness, or anaesthetize her against anger, grief, and anxiety. It may even become a best friend, one that is always available (Miller, 1994).

I went through a phase where I wanted to harm myself. I felt worthless so why didn't I just take it one step further to the point of ridding myself. What was going through my mind is no one will know this. When I was fourteen or fifteen and in high school that went through my mind. Obviously I didn't know how to cope. The nurturing wasn't there. Some friends had rejected me and I felt abandoned. I was thrown into this state by what had happened. I made a pact with myself that if things didn't get better in a year I would kill myself, but of course I forgot about that three months later.

*Lisa*

Remembering the past, and grieving those life experiences that have been denied or those that have vanished, the mother-daughter incest survivor may at times be overwhelmed by waves of anger that rush over her. She may be left with a burden of unexpressed rage against those who remained indifferent to her fate and who failed to help or protect her. Rage outbursts further perpetuate her isolation and prevent the restoration or establishment of relationships. The survivor may attempt to control her rage by withdrawing from other people or directing her rage and hatred against herself.

> The rage is tied up with the grief which is tied up with the memory, and a lot of body stuff. Digestive system, migraine headaches, a lot of stuff tied to the abuse. I have to dissociate. I carry it in my body. I have problems in my lower back, and I know it's related to my mother. I tell myself I was bad and dirty, untouchable and unlovable. I carry the abuse experience with me in terms of how I relate to myself. It is not in a very positive manner. I have low self-esteem, a lot of issues around relationships. I have a lot of stuff around being bad. The guilt really affects me. I know that I have been told and I have experienced it as well that I am an extremely competent person in my field in music and art as well. It doesn't match, though, with what I feel inside. There is a huge discrepancy. My core belief of myself has been affected, and this affects my quality of life, my inner peace and happiness. My friends tell me who I am and how wonderful I am. I hear them but it still does not match up with what's inside at my core.
>
> *Mable*

It is important for the helping professional to be aware that mother-daughter incest survivors are adept at "tuning out and turning off." Not unlike other abuse survivors, tuning in to feelings is frightening for them. They have tremendous fear about losing control. They are afraid that talking about the abuse will force them to relive it and render them out of control all over again. Feeling safe may be synonymous with being in control. Maintaining control for her may mean perfectionism or being perfect. Being perfect may mean greatness, popularity, not being vulnerable, and having friends flock to her. Throughout the process of therapy, the survivor may question how to be perfect. She may decide that being better means being vulnerable, honest, and willing to experience emotions and pain. On the other hand, she may be repulsed by her vulnerability (Rhodes and Rhodes, 1996).

The mother-daughter incest survivor may be left feeling a tremendous push from an unseen force that has the potential to erase or annihilate her from the universe. She fears that once again her sense of existence and belonging will be denied, that she doesn't have a secure position, a rightful place in humanity or in the scheme of things. Many survivors find themselves unconsciously attracted to that which they fear the most. Essentially what they resist, persists. They are drawn to people who are hostile and domineering because they pattern choices after the past. Recognizing this pattern is helpful for the client; seeing is freeing.

> I've gone through disastrous relationships. I remember having no self-esteem and so I made lousy choices. I was so naive, and my self-worth and self-respect were in the collective toilet. I'm still certainly struggling with it. I'm trying to transcend the legacy she left me, of self-abuse. What happens is that you put yourself in situations where this person is going to manipulate you or control you, like mother did, or take advantage of you or whatever.

> *Alana*

For many survivors of mother-daughter incest, a tremendous fear exists that their mother is still going to get them. Many women fear that their mothers are just roaming around ready to pounce. They still carry memories as a child of mother being superhuman and limitless in terms of what she could do to them. Some survivors fear that even after death their mother could become more powerful and continue to murder their soul, dash their hopes, and turn their dreams into nightmares.

The emotional state of the mother-daughter incest survivor, like that of other chronically abused children, ranges from a baseline of unease, through intermediate states of anxiety and dysphoria, to extremes of panic, fury, and despair. Not surprisingly, a great many survivors develop chronic anxiety and depression which persist into adulthood.

I feel like I'm going through a breakdown. I've been depressed
for years and years. It's so hard not to surrender, for that would
mean admitting that I am a failure, not strong enough, that
something is wrong with me. I feel I should be able to get
through this. I should be stronger. I should be able to handle it
all. I feel like she's won. I have a difficult time not seeing myself
as being very damaged. I don't know if anyone will ever love
me. I'm beyond hope of having anything normal in terms of relationships, children. I have a hard time standing up for myself,
to say no. I have a hard time being myself because I still don't
know who that is. With women, I don't feel safe. I hate women.
That's hard to explain to a woman. I go through such hatred and
rage but I don't want to. I don't want to hate women because that
would mean that I hate myself. I feel so ashamed because I don't
know what to do about it.

*Sonia*

Purging and vomiting, compulsive sexual behavior, compulsive risk
taking or exposure to danger, and use of psychoactive drugs become
vehicles by which the mother-daughter incest survivor attempts to
regulate her internal emotional states. It is vitally important that the
therapist acknowledge that as a survivor of prolonged repeated childhood trauma, the mother-daughter incest survivor may become a danger
to herself. Possible sources of danger may include self-harm, passive
failures of self-protection, and pathological dependency on the abuser.

The mother-daughter incest survivor will need to create an internal
nurturing parent. It may be important for her to reparent and soothe
the inner child, and separate that inner child from her adult self, to become whole and competent. It is essential that the mother-daughter
incest survivor recognize that she can be a competent adult, that she
has the power to take control of her life, take care of herself, and experience self-mastery. No longer should her mother control her. Part
of her learning process will involve learning techniques to enable her
to take charge of her feelings. The therapist will need to reinforce that
she is an adult, not a child anymore, and therefore in a better position
to deal with emotions and fears in a positive, action-oriented fashion.
The adult mother-daughter incest survivor has the chance to get to
know herself and to be totally honest about her feelings and emotions.

I didn't know what it was to have feelings. I didn't know what anger was. I was pretty out to lunch. I still remember picking my daughter up when she was about three-and-a-half, and I was just going to throw her against the wall and I saw her face and it stopped me. I wasn't aware I was angry. When I saw her eyes I knew I was acting out what had been done to me. Then it shook me up. It made me watch myself more, to really care for her.

*Michelle*

Seeing a therapist, reading, journaling, rewriting old rules and values that keep her trapped, soliciting the support of family members and friends, writing about dreams, and using guided imagery represent ways that the mother-daughter incest survivor can take charge of her life. They represent constructive strategies to help her to taste freedom, recharge her psychic batteries, bring happiness into her life, and give her the strength to persevere.

In order to take charge of her own self-care, the mother-daughter incest survivor must regain the ability to take initiative, carry out plans, and exercise independent judgment. The capacities for self-care and self-soothing, which could not develop in childhood, must be painstakingly constructed in later life. As she begins to exercise these capabilities, which have been undermined by repeated childhood abuse, she enhances her sense of competence, self-esteem, and power, and begins to take control of the decision-making process. She can also be encouraged to confront her old family blueprint and to make significant changes in beliefs, rules, values, and attitudes that she learned as a child that no longer are congruent with who she is today. She can examine these rules, accept some, reject others, and rewrite the ones she confutes. By figuring out what her family's attitudes were toward play, work, women, sex, marriage, etc., she will discover the inner core of her family's belief system. She can challenge in great depth her family's philosophy of life and become active to create a more positive life for herself. She can create her own personal constitution or blueprint which will be an affirmation of herself and her life (Kunzman, 1990).

In summary, mother-daughter incest survivors carry profound feelings of guilt, of being tainted by their abuse experience. They bury their deep secret within their minds. For most adult survivors, the combination of sexual abuse, the secrecy surrounding it, and the phenomenal isolation and shame they feel continues to cause great stress in their lives. It forces them to suppress or deny their feelings, to have their voices muted. It colors their present-day life and squashes any hope for the future. Breaking the silence and dismantling the wall of secrecy is the first and most important step to recovery. For the mother-daughter incest survivor this becomes a phenomenal leap, a huge risk, and a horrifying venture into a place that is often met with personal and societal denial of the existence of the phenomenon of mother-daughter incest.

The therapist must be committed to the client's goals, and to respect her coping strategies. It is the responsibility of the therapist to secure a safe environment that requires attention not only to the client's psychological capacity to protect herself but also to the realities of power in her social situation. She will need a safe environment to progress to the next stages of recovery, which involves in-depth exploration of the traumatic abuse experience at the hands of her mother (Epstein, 1994). The therapist will need to reactivate the client's blocked learning processes, so that the client can develop new coping strategies to reach her goals (Miltenburg and Singer, 1997). Therapeutic interventions will need to be developed by encouraging the survivor to learn new ways of coping in the world, to develop her own interests and talents. The therapist must recognize that the mother-daughter incest survivor will need time to gradually emerge from the burden of pain, isolation, and shame. With help, she can learn new growth responses, such as problem-solving skills, healthy strategies for mind and body, and resolution of her anger. She can overcome her fear and desire to distance herself or to engage in self-injurious behavior. She no longer will need to stay distant and suspicious of other people, in particular, other women. Through understanding what happened to her in childhood, she will grow to accept that she was blameless regarding her childhood abuse and that she is an adult now capable of assuming power. Once she clearly sees that the abuse is a comment on her mother, and not on herself or all women, she will be enabled to experience real intimacy in healthy relationships. Over time, stressful and regressive episodes for the client will diminish such that she will not be incapacitated by fear and anxiety. She can then be freed from the tyranny of her past.

# *PART III:*
# *COMMON THEMES*
# *AMONG MOTHERS*

Although the emphasis of the interviews with the women was on their own experience of abuse at the hands of their mothers, they commonly, throughout the study, described their mothers as:

1. emotionally needy and unstable; and
2. committing boundary violations.

This section of the book addresses these themes from the daughter's perspective and incorporates therapeutic interventions. Further research is necessary to address a mother's motivation for perpetrating the sexual abuse of her daughter.

# Chapter 9

# Emotionally Needy
# and Unstable Mothers

By the time I was thirteen the role reversal was complete. Mom
was dependent on me, and I was stronger than her. She was forever trying to cry on my shoulder. What was most difficult for
me was that she was so weak and dependent, which forced me
into this role reversal. I get my back up whenever I'm around
women who I perceive as being needy or manipulating.

*Sue*

Victims of mother-daughter incest are clearly from fractured families that are unable to provide fundamental emotional development
for their members. The mothers in these families fail to provide
nurturance and safety for their children. Mother-daughter incest survivors have been inadequately parented and their needs as children
were sacrificed for those of their mothers. They are left feeling that
their mothers were deficient and defective in their mothering role.

Many mother-daughter incest survivors experience their mothers
as lonely, miserable, and isolated. They often report that their mothers are insecure, inadequate, unstable, and unempathic. They perceive their mothers as having extreme needs for intimacy, attention,
and affection. Many survivors believe that their mothers rely on them
for emotional support. They speak of their mothers' instability, dependence, and unsettledness, and as having marked difficulties in
psychological and social functioning.

She couldn't keep friends. She rotated through them. People
soon figured out that she was unpredictable and unstable. She
would accuse people of things that didn't happen. She was so
mean and vindictive, yet on a good day she could be like a nor-

mal mom. You wouldn't know, though, when that was going to be, so there was always a lot of stress. I would be really worried and scared and extremely ill when she would visit. That was so confusing for me, and that's why I'd get sick before seeing her and after seeing her. Three days after I'd still be bedridden.

*Ashley*

I attempted to have her institutionalized for her own sake because she was suicidal. She would slit her wrists. She would call me from phone booths when I was a child to say that she had slit her wrist and that she was at a phone booth, that she was about to bleed to death. It's all my fault. I would be forced to attempt to find out where she was. It sounds insane even talking about it. It sounds so bizarre. It seems like somebody else's life in retrospect. I've sort of disassociated myself from everything.

*Alana*

Victims of mother-daughter incest often describe their mothers as extremely volatile, as capable of switching instantly from normal to violent and back.

It was like living with Dr. Jekyll and Mrs. Hyde. I never knew from one minute to the next when I was growing up what she was going to be like. I'd remember always feeling hostile toward her and afraid because she was so volatile all the time. You never knew when she was going to erupt.

*Iris*

These mothers may portray the helpless victim role, claiming they have been victimized by their children or their husbands. For these abusive mothers, this serves the purpose of gathering sympathy and attention from significant others, and from people around them who, as members of society, naturally want to protect mothers.

I felt that my mother's happiness was my responsibility. She was very much the martyr, very much the victim. My dad is an alcoholic and she gets a lot of attention. People pity her. She plays the wounded-bird role well. She's very good at that. The perception that I had was that people thought she was a good mother. After all, we were always clean, our hair was always combed, we had nice clothes. When the doors were closed though, my mom was very cold. The hardest part for me is that everybody thought that she was a great mom. I felt that I could not disclose that she wasn't that way at all, but that she was a fraud and abusive. I felt that I really took it on as it must be me, there must be something wrong with me because every other mother seems to be warm. I saw her being warm with other little girls so it must be me, there's something inherently wrong with me. It made me feel so crazy because no one else could see her for what she really was. She was so cold to me. I grew up with the feeling that she hated me. I didn't understand why. I just thought that I wasn't good enough. As a kid, I felt ignored and rejected, pushed aside. Somewhere in me I knew I would never be good enough for her to love, so there was no point in me trying.

*Sonia*

My mother spent time in psychiatric hospitals. She had mental problems. I think she may have been schizophrenic. She tried to keep up the facade of being the good housekeeper, though. I don't know how people viewed her because she had breakdowns. I think people felt sorry for her. She played the victim quite often. My father certainly would feel sorry for her. I guess I was expected to be her mother in a sense. She expected me to have all the answers.

*Michelle*

Many survivors perceive their mothers as constantly endeavoring to display and preserve their feminine image, as feeling strongly they had to protect it. This feminine image, as defined by society, sets up the notion that motherhood is next to godliness, that it is sainthood and that mothers do not perpetrate acts of violence. For mothers who are coperpetrators, being feminine perhaps means being passive, unassertive, supportive, and protective of their husbands who are also perpetrating. When the mother co-offends with her spouse, her dependency on him may be a major contributing factor and when she independently offends, her need for nurturance and control appear prominent (McCarthy, 1986).

From a feminist perspective, social conditions create and perpetuate the pattern that women are underrepresented, devalued, disempowered in every aspect of society, and treated as second-class citizens. These myths are generated and perpetuated by the dominant group culture which takes shape and form from a patriarchal society. As a result, many women suffer privately with their anger and dissatisfaction, feel powerless and helpless, and stuck in their relationships. They may act out their frustration and rage on their children.

Many survivors of maternal incest describe their mothers as having a strong fear of abandonment. This reinforces their need to protect their spouses and not confront them about their perpetration and their physical and emotional absence. Some mothers are abuse victims themselves; some have been sexually abused as children; some are physically battered by their husbands. Neediness may cause them to feel overwhelmed and perhaps resentful of their child's needs. They may be too angry, too bitter, too pained, and too confused to give out any kind of love to their children. They may abuse their daughters to express hostility or self-hatred. They may work long hours, be chronically ill, or overinvolved with household chores. They may be absent emotionally. If they had been sexually abused in childhood by their mothers, they may be replicating their own abuse experience with their daughters. As a result, they struggle more with developing a relationship with their own daughter. They may hate or resent their femaleness.

Matthews and colleagues (1991) studied sixteen females who were referred to the Genesis Female Sexual Offenders Treatment Program in Minnesota. Nine of the women described themselves as needing acceptance, attention, and closeness, as having unmet needs or low self-esteem, and feeling isolated. Feelings of anger, revenge, power, jealousy, and rejection were listed by seven women as reasons for their abusive behavior. The majority reported that their children were safe targets for these displaced feelings. Four of the women believed their acts were expressions of love, either for the victim or the husband.

I just feel like she treated me like this human garbage can. She couldn't deal with her anger, rage, whatever she was feeling.

The fact that she was married to someone so she had to submit or she had to sleep with him. She couldn't deal with that so she turned around and took it all out on me. All her feelings she couldn't deal with were dumped so I had to take them on because I was so young that I didn't know any better. I just feel this strong enmeshment. She cuts her finger and I feel the pain.

*Sonia*

Mothers may experience a great deal of internal conflict often stimulated by their role as mother, in particular, if memories of unresolved wishes from their own infancy are evoked. Mothers may be parasitic, that is, they may relive their own infancy through their daughters. They may hold onto their daughters because they have little else in their lives, nothing of their own. They may be so frustrated in their relationships with their own mothers that they try to make up for it through symbiosis with their daughters. Some mothers try to fill up the empty hole inside left by their own cold, distant, abusive, or absent mother by merging with their daughters. They may want their daughters to be the other half of them, the warm extension they long for. These mothers may insist that their daughters tell them everything about their lives and their friends. They may become over-interested, curious, or obsessed with their daughters sexuality. Boundary violations often result from the mother's possession of their daughters and from their perceptions that their daughters are extensions of themselves and not separate persons. This may awaken in the mother the part of her that feels needy and wants to be nurtured and responded to. As an abused child she may display a strong picture of frozen watchfulness toward her mother, hyper alert for what might happen. She may at times show an unusual sensitivity to the needs and wants of her mother. She may have learned early that it is possible to placate a disturbed and potentially abusive mother by constantly attending to her wishes.

The repressed little girl inside mother often shapes the mother-daughter relationship. The mother may act toward her daughter in the same way she acts internally toward the little girl part of herself. The daughter becomes an external representation of that part of herself she has come to deny, dislike, or blame. Complex emotions from the mother's own childhood deprivation and adult life may be directed inward to negate the little girl part of herself and outward onto her daughter. In a sense, the mother, through her daughter, lives both her own childhood and her own mother's identity. By identifying with her daughter, she becomes both her own mother and her own child.

Mothers, deprived of love in their childhood, may seek from their daughters the love they lacked from their mothers. In doing so, they are inverting the normal parent-child relationship, requiring their daughters to act as parents while they become children.

> I ended up being the caretaker, and I think that's just one of the reasons I have this incredible memory that goes back further. I ended up being the one who took care of things, who took charge. If anything got done, I was the one who did it. From the time I was ten, my mother would retreat into her own times because of her mental illness. I would take over and do the housework. I was always the one who was responsible and kept everything going.
>
> *Arabella*

This places tremendous burden on the daughters with huge expectations to comply and show gratitude for the care they receive. In conforming to their mothers' wishes, they build up a one-sided picture of their mothers as wholly loving and generous, thereby shutting out from consciousness much information reaching them that their mothers are selfish, demanding, and ungrateful. They may only allow into their consciousness feelings of love and gratitude for their mothers while repressing feelings of anger they may have against their mothers for expecting them to be caregivers while not noticing the demands being made of them. This prevents them from making friends and living their own life.

> I know she doesn't like it that I'm so close to my roommate. She'll often say, "I think you like your friends better than you like me." I feel like saying it's true. She's always portrayed herself as Little Orphan Annie. I guess I see her as a needy, clingy, lonely kid. Just needy, not pathological or psychotic. I felt like I betrayed her by leaving her. She needed me to stay there. It was like my job to stay there and take care of her. I betrayed her by leaving home. When she came out to visit me a little while ago, she followed me everywhere. I'd go to work, and she'd want to drive to work with me. She'd go shopping, meet me for lunch,

and be there after work. She was everywhere all the time. I'd go into my room to change and she'd follow me in. I'd have to go to the bathroom and shut the door. It's just like Velcro.

*Jan*

Role reversal may be a strong element in mother-daughter incestuous relationships. The mother who had unsatisfactory mothering may look for love and mothering from the young daughter who cannot meet these expectations. This may engender rage in the mother and re-awaken earlier deprivation and loss from her own childhood. Mothers may place high expectations on their daughters in terms of meeting their nurturance needs. In essence, the daughter assumes the maternal role. When mothers turn to their daughters for emotional nurturance, the effect may be a total role reversal in their relationship. In some instances, an older daughter may serve as a surrogate partner for the mother, often having adult responsibilities. In cases where mothers project a more controlling, hostile, or sadistic personality, the daughter may serve as the object of her mother's intrusive, exploratory, and sometimes sadistic sexual contact.

In summary, the clinician must be aware that a mother may herself have been a victim of childhood incest with her father or mother and may therefore believe that repetition of this phenomenon is acceptable. She may even be an accomplice to an incestuous relationship between her husband and her daughter. Incestuous mothers, similar to perpetrators of other forms of sexual abuse, are often products of physically abusive or neglectful families. They may perceive themselves as being ineffective with their peer group. They may feel out of control, and that those who have control are powerful. To feel powerful and to achieve control they may turn to others less powerful. They may offend because they feel that control can only be achieved through victimization of others. Whatever the reason women sexually abuse their daughters, they abandon their maternal role for an exploitive relationship with their daughter. The daughters are left feeling that they have been sacrificed in order to satisfy or care for their mothers.

It was so painful for me because it was so one-sided. It was so strange, such a parasitical relationship. She expected me to be her savior. My relationship with her was so bad that when I was raped my mother had the nerve, the audacity, to tell me that it was my fault, and that I deserved it. That is how grossly insensitive this woman was. If she could have stolen something from me that I needed, she would have done it. She hated me. That was the worst part, to be hated by your mother. She felt a real desire to absolutely squash my happiness, to alienate any signs of happiness in my life. She constantly denigrated my choices in life. I wasn't allowed to have boyfriends. I wasn't allowed to have friends. I was allowed to work, though, because she got the money from that so that was acceptable to her. Even then, she felt that I was having too much fun at work.

*Alana*

# Chapter 10

# Boundary Violations

The sexual abuse I can remember. She would come back from going out to bars, and she would take me to the bedroom and use me to masturbate with. I can remember her pushing my face into her genitals.

*Alice*

All children need consistent safety and trust to feel secure. It is a child's right to be cared for and shielded from violence, to have a life free from adult sexuality, and to have a positive identity. Mother-daughter incest survivors, to the contrary, received incredible personal violation at the hands of their mothers. Their rights were stolen from them by the very person who was supposed to protect them. They were invaded, offended, and intruded upon by their mothers. As children, they were neglected, disrespected, and hurt when their basic rights to be protected, nurtured, and guided were violated. The mother-daughter incest survivor, in particular, feels violated because she was abused by the one person closest to her. Her mother robbed her of her childhood, her innocence, her ownership of her body, and her sexuality. This damaged trust and disrupted bonding.

Her abusing me at age four sort of severed the bonds that were there. You lose trust. You don't know what's going to happen next. Still at age thirty-three, I'm in that position of not knowing what's going to happen next. I don't trust her. I don't know what she's going to do next to hurt me. It's just the way I am every day, wondering what she is going to do next.

*Jacqueline*

The mother-daughter incest survivor is abused by her mother in overt, perhaps extreme ways, or through covert means that may be verbal in nature or under the guise of hygiene or protection. Her mother may administer excessive enemas that not only purge her body but also her mind. The perpetrator may be sadistically attempting to rid her body of the devil; perhaps she believes that cleanliness is next to godliness. Her mother may roughly rub or scrub her daughter's genitals to the point of rawness and pain. She might regularly examine her daughter's underpants to see if she can find evidence of her daughter's sexual activity. Blatant cruelty may occur, such as penetration with implements, torture and burning of genitals, being held under water until near drowning, being locked in attics, basements, or dark closets, or being physically punched, kicked, or beaten with an assortment of weapons. A wide variety of overt and covert sexual behaviors may occur ranging from voyeurism, exploitation, kissing, and fondling, to oral sex, digital penetration, and penetration by implements.

> My mom was so inappropriate a lot of the time when it came to being affectionate. She'd like to kiss me on the lips.
>
> *Ashley*

Whatever is done to the victim, it is destruction of the body and the soul. The mother-daughter incest survivor may not be allowed to show emotion or to express pain. Life for her is often inescapably bound up in secrecy. The threat of violence is often present during childhood for victims of mother-daughter incest. They may constantly feel physically, emotionally, and sexually threatened. Threats of harm by their mothers ensure secrecy; hence, these women live in social isolation enforced by their mothers. Although they are violated in varying degrees by their mothers, the grave consequences of their violation impacts them developmentally throughout their lives. As children, they carry the secret of their abuse into adulthood, leaving them with conflicts that affect their daily functioning.

> She chipped away at my self-esteem. I was always stupid, an idiot, a slut, a tart. I don't even remember how she came up with the terms, but certainly she seemed to have a full arsenal of those. She would berate me constantly. Nothing was ever good

enough. If I washed the floor, she'd get mad because it wasn't good enough. She'd hit me because she didn't like the way I set the table. I can remember one time she chased me with a knife. I was in the middle of stuffing a chicken. I had tied it up very nicely. She didn't like it, and so she started hitting me and chasing me around the living room/dining room. Two of my friends were coming up the driveway and actually saw her chasing me with the knife. After that, they started to believe what was going on in my house. Up until then, I appeared to be so normal that no one really understood what was really going on. You would not believe the things I had to go through. It was horrible. She would tell me that if it wasn't for me, her marriage would have been better. She would tell me her marriage wasn't going well and it was all my fault. She wished I had never been born and she hated me, and if I would leave everything would be better. I was the source of all her troubles. The sexual stuff was really hard for me to sort out. It took me years to take a look at it. I remembered very clearly having a black item, I think it was a thermometer case, inserted into my vagina, when I was very, very young. I can remember quite often having severe vaginal infections, redness, and soreness. It hurt to pass water. It scared me, and I would use a lot of creams and things in order to be able to wear underpants and that sort of thing.

*Alana*

The issue of sexual abuse by one's mother is complicated. As a young child, one's mother was turned to in times of need. The adult survivor may express grief and confusion and question her mother's motives, e.g., "How could she do that to me? She's like me. We're both female." The uniqueness of the situation contributes to the survivor's feelings of alienation, isolation, self-doubt, self-blame, and low self-esteem.

Mother-daughter incest survivors grieve and feel depressed over the loss of their most trusted figure. They believe that because they experienced disconnection, boundary violations, and sexual abuse at the hands of their mothers, somehow they are less worthy of respect, particularly damaged and reprehensible, and even deserving of further victimization. Developing trust, of believing in themselves and in others, is an extremely difficult issue for mother-daughter incest survivors. Many survivors feel stalked and unsafe continually in their daily lives. The impact of this mistrust is phenomenal in terms of how it contributes to isolation and aversion to intimacy. They are afraid to develop close relationships with anyone. They fear sexual involvement because their mother used sex as a form of abuse.

Mother-daughter incest survivors may find themselves in extremely vulnerable positions time and time again because they have not been taught safety, and have come from an incestuous family where boundaries are too rigid or too permeable. Mothers, particularly if they are abuse victims themselves, may struggle with loose boundaries and an inadequate sense of self. They may become overwhelmingly enmeshed with their daughters such that they do not know where they end and their daughters begin. This dynamic may set the stage for the exceptionally needy mother to cross physical, emotional, and sexual boundaries, to subtlely seduce her daughter without fear of detection.

The child who is subjected to excessive invasion of privacy by her mother or other adult family members may respond with secrecy to this violation. The practitioner needs to understand that refusing to disclose or to share information may be an attempt by the victim to retain some form of control, to establish some semblance of longed-for privacy. When the victims are young, the practitioner needs to be aware that grave disenchantment and disillusionment may lead the child to an intense need to regain trust and security, or become manifested in extreme dependency and clinging. Anger stemming from betrayal may be behind the aggressive and hostile stance that these women may take as adolescents.

It is not uncommon for the mother-daughter incest survivor to engage in or even invent crises and chaos as a way to feel loved and needed. She may fall into a pattern of connecting with others through the intensity of chaos and abuse. The therapist can assist the client to distinguish between legitimate concerns and concerns that are the responsibility of others. The client can be encouraged to make decisions about herself and to experience self-possession. Once the client knows herself better, she will come to realize that she has much to offer and something to give. She can be comfortable with other people. She can know the joy of intimacy. Learning to trust her own decisions and her own intuition will inevitably decrease her feelings of powerlessness, helplessness, and anxiety. She will be less likely to lose herself in a relationship or to isolate herself to avoid interpersonal connections.

Given the fact that the mother-daughter incest survivor experienced boundary violations by her mother, it will be critical for the therapist to pay particular attention to the establishment and maintenance of clear boundaries within the therapeutic alliance such that the client does not face further violation. The lack of clearly drawn boundaries almost always exists in the life of a mother-daughter incest survivor. She will need to understand that it is essential for her to become secure about personal boundaries and develop the courage and strength to enforce them. The practitioner will need to encourage her to set boundaries that will allow her to feel safe in the world and to say no if she is threatened in any way.

> I'm afraid that if I have a close relationship with someone, issues will come up. Chances are good that more issues will start to emerge with friends. I'll start to have difficulty with my female relationships. I'm afraid that issues will be compounded with a woman. In relationships with men, it is easier for me to keep boundaries.
>
> *Mable*

The therapist must encourage the client to strive toward meeting caring people through safe, healthy avenues, to avoid situations and relationships that are threatening and intrusive, while seeking those that feel safe and supportive. Through group therapy, the client can experience what a safe environment is like, where members are respected and protected. Joining a group can be one of the best and most constructive ways for the mother-daughter incest survivor to take a giant leap forward on the road to recovery. The group has built-in safety features such as a professionally trained facilitator, a structured setting, and group rules that protect members. Structured support from group members allows for feedback which will be especially helpful when dealing with frightening feelings. The group can re-create some of the positive family dynamics that members missed in their families of origin. The group will disallow abusive behavior, and the mother-daughter incest survivor will be encouraged to discuss her feelings. Furthermore, the group can provide a great place to give and receive caring touches and hugs, which can be very healing for the mother-daughter incest survivor. Within the group, she can find hope, connect with others, and come to accept and care for herself as a worthwhile person.

Finally, the practitioner will need to acknowledge the existence of diffuse boundaries between mothers and daughters and that a less separate sense of self is a cultural phenomenon, sanctioned by society. It is important to note, however, that because their mothers had poor boundaries themselves, it was difficult for the daughters to learn that they had distinct boundaries. For some of these women, the effect of mother-daughter incest has been so deep that they may struggle with mothering their own children. They may experience difficulty in their mothering role, particularly in terms of establishing boundaries. They may even cross the line with their own children and commit boundary violations. The clinician must check to see if the mother-daughter incest survivor, who is a mother herself, has victimized her child in any way. The clinician must be ready to ask the survivor if she has sexually abused her child, or if she has fantasized about perpetrating against her child. Therapy can assist the client in establishing and maintaining boundaries between herself and her children as well as other significant people in her life.

> What worked for me in therapy was my therapist always believed me, even when I was having doubts. She was my strength. She never crowded me or tried to touch me but instead really kept a distance. I'd never known that I had a right to my own space. I learned that from her. I learned in therapy that I didn't like people being very close to me. I learned to ask for distance and space and to be okay with it. I learned that to need space is not a shameful or awful thing or a big defect. It's the way I am and it's okay. My therapist modeled for me what an appropriate relationship can be. She let me establish boundaries and she respected them. I felt in control for the first time. I had never had that kind of power or control. I could even refuse to do anything my therapist suggested. It's all up to me. I was blessed to find a caring and nurturing therapist. When I need to be a child, very young and dependent, she's there. I don't allow myself to be

very dependent because it's so threatening. I feel so safe with her. She'll hold me if I ask her to. I've even gotten angry with her, and I'm not the greatest at expressing my anger. It doesn't always come out in a nice therapeutic way, but she still likes me.

*Sonia*

# PART IV:
# SPECIFIC COUNSELING
# INTERVENTIONS

Unique counseling issues specific to the phenomenon of mother-daughter incest will need to be addressed in therapy for mother-daughter incest survivors. Although this form of abuse is rare, the limited empirical evidence indicates that the experience and consequences of this abuse are quite profound, with implications that extend far and deep into the lives of survivors. Maternal abuse survivors reportedly benefit from many of the therapeutic interventions that are commonly utilized when working with survivors of paternal abuse, particularly interventions focused on alleviating their feelings of self-blame, guilt, lack of trust, and shame. However, the following salient counseling issues will be given particular attention in this part of the book: (1) stigmatization; (2) identity development; (3) parenting; and (4) treating the adult victim. These issues differentiate mother-daughter incest victims from other victims of sexual abuse and make their experience more unique. Counseling interventions to assist practitioners with these issues will be addressed, along with some strategies for victims of mother-daughter incest who continue to be victimized into adulthood by their mothers.

# Chapter 11

# Stigmatization

I feel overwhelmed by intense feelings of guilt, shame, and despair. This reinforces my experience of profound isolation. I'm so frightened by the thought that my experience does not match that of others.

*Patti*

Shame has been a huge issue for me. I'm not aware of what I feel. I'm much more aware than I've ever been now. I do know what I was experiencing was shame. I didn't know they were feelings. I didn't know I had feelings. I have to unlock my behavior. I know I feel a tremendous amount of shame. I remember talking to a friend something about my mother trying to kill me and sexually abusing me. She couldn't handle it. It sort of reinforced the shame that I had. People don't like to hear things that they can't handle. I have the feeling that I'm defective or flawed. I was always feeling ashamed of how I was and how I am. I've felt defective from the start.

*Michelle*

It is imperative that the helping professional be receptive to the fact that the shame of mother-daughter incest is more profound and the stigmatization more extreme because the abuse experience is in the minority among all forms of child abuse. Mother-daughter incest is the least understood of all types of sexual abuse and is the final type of incest to be investigated.

The mother-daughter incest survivor feels isolated and alienated from the world because she believes she is different from everyone else and that her abuse experience is "out of the ordinary." Hence, she feels reluctant to disclose that her mother was her abuser. The helping professional must be open to the possibility that a mother-daughter incest survivor may present with issues regarding paternal incest, when in reality her mother perpetrated the abuse. The survivor may experience difficulty with labeling her abuse as mother-daughter incest.

> As intellectual as I am, I didn't know the name mother-daughter incest existed, which is really funny because I spent my life in it.

> *Patti*

The practitioner must attempt to understand and respect the client's position. The shame and stigma the client feels as a result of her abuse may contribute to her reluctance to disclose or accept that her mother was her abuser. Shame forces the mother-daughter incest survivor into silence and draws her into a world of secrecy. Shame is a predominant feature in her psychological landscape. Because her mother was her abuser, she feels tremendous self-blame and responsibility for the abuse.

As with other severely shamed people, the mother-daughter incest survivor may project her own feelings onto other people, incorrectly assuming that all humans have the same viewpoint. Since mother-daughter incest survivors despise themselves, they believe that everyone else detests them as well. Their self-denigration is so profound that they find it impossible to receive respect and affection from others. This self-deprecation and self-condemnation, along with negative self-talk, reinforces their shame.

Due to the stigma and isolation she feels, she may abuse drugs and alcohol, attempt suicide, or commit other self-destructive acts. Because shame originates in early childhood for the mother-daughter incest survivor, avoidance tends to become the norm. Avoidance inhibits social experiences and the development of social skills, hence social experiences are not successful. The downward spiral continues, encouraging further avoidance and cultivating the survivor's enduring inability to form attachments and become intimate. When relationships do form, they are typically superficial in nature (Brassell, 1994).

The restoration of social bonds begins with the discovery that one is not alone. Nowhere is this experience more immediate, powerful, or convincing than in a group. The therapeutic impact of universality is particularly significant for the mother-daughter incest survivor who has felt phenomenal isolation and stigma by her shameful secret. Groups for the mother-daughter incest survivor play a special role in her recovery process in that she receives a degree of support and understanding, a feeling of acceptance, that is absent in her world. The group provides the survivor with the opportunity to engage in a meaningful social connection, with mutually enhancing interactions, rewarding relationships, and the experience of collective empowerment. Members discover that interconnection with others is a critical aspect of healing. Group members approach one another as peers and equals. They are able to draw upon the shared resources of the group to foster their recovery (Herman, 1992; Knight, 1997).

> I completed two sessions of four months each, very intensive anger work. It was excruciating, but it saved my life. The group treatment was excellent. We had the same symptoms. There was one other person who had been abused by her grandmother. We talked about how we all had the same aftereffects, and I had a difficult time with older women at that time. I had such fear of older women—that they were untrustworthy and unreliable.

*Ashley*

Group therapy can be a particularly significant and helpful form of therapy since it provides the context for reworking the impaired interpersonal functioning and mistrust which resulted from the trauma of the abuse experience. Group therapy encourages breaking of the silence. Encountering others who have undergone similar experiences dissolves feelings of isolation, shame, and stigma for the mother-daughter incest survivor. It allows her to connect to others and express her individuality in a controlled healing environment. The group understands her fluctuating need for closeness and distance. They relate to her profound need to establish autonomy and control. Because group members experience similar challenges in their lives, they are more sympathetic and understanding. They do not judge her. They give her permission to express her feelings and overcome her feelings of shame and self-blame. Sharing her abuse experience with others who have experienced the same is a "precondition for the restitution of a sense of a meaningful world" (Herman, 1992, p. 70).

Group therapy has really worked—being with other women who have been in the same situation. I did a ten-week group and somebody brought up the topic of cutting. It was the best day I'd had in months. Somebody else did exactly the same things as me. I wasn't nuts. I was able to communicate with group members because I had something in common. It was great that there was somebody to link up with. And that makes individual counseling easier. So it helped me big time knowing that there were people out there and that you weren't alone.

*Elsie*

Group members often become substitute parents and siblings (Brassell, 1994). Group therapy provides a safe and consistent environment for sharing and empathy in which survivors can explore their reactions to their abuse and the effect of the abuse experience in their daily lives. New skills and behaviors are developed and rehearsed which help group members undo the damage from the abuse. Typical group themes may include experiences of loss and rage, self-doubt and self-blame, feeling responsible for their abuse, shame, isolation, and stigma.

At the beginning, I didn't even know what I was feeling. I had gone to group therapy for about ten months, and each week you go in you talk about how you are feeling. I hadn't a damn clue what I felt. I couldn't put a name to what I was feeling. Over time, it progresses. Now I pretty much know what I'm feeling.

*Sonia*

The dynamics of the group and the interplay of group members may help the mother-daughter incest survivor examine her reaction to other group members and uncover social interaction problems that might not be so readily apparent in individual counseling. She can learn the skill of assertiveness, which is a major strategy for overcoming loneliness. She will practice better communication skills and through assertiveness she will become more honest and forthright about her interests, her ways of doing things, her feelings, her likes and dislikes (Gil, 1996). She builds a sense of basic safety and a positive view of herself and the world.

The therapist may encourage the mother-daughter incest survivor to

> involve herself in social action, drawing upon her own initiative, energy and resourcefulness, and magnifying these qualities far beyond her own capabilities. Involving herself in organized, demanding social efforts based on cooperation and shared purpose challenges her to call upon her most mature, adaptive coping strategies of patience, anticipation, altruism, and humor. Social action will bring out the best in her, while allowing her the sense of connection with the best in other people. She may choose to focus her energies on helping others who have been similarly victimized, on educational, legal, or political efforts to prevent victimization of others. (Herman, 1992, p. 207)

Finally, the practitioner must provide a safe environment wherein survivors of maternal incest can acknowledge that mothers are not omnipotent, selfless creatures who are beyond behaving in ways that are damaging to their children. Acknowledging and contextualizing their experiences will help reduce acute feelings of stigmatization for mother-daughter incest survivors, legitimize and validate their feelings and experiences, and assist them to recognize that they were not responsible for the abuse. Early child work may be particularly helpful in assisting the client to acknowledge her powerlessness in stopping the abuse and in normalizing her feelings of shame and guilt.

The therapist plays a key role in convincing the mother-daughter incest survivor that she will need to push shame aside and replace it with such positive attributes as dignity, self-worth, and admiration for her successes. The therapist can encourage her to learn thought patterns to guide her emotions and behaviors, overcome loneliness, and control her fear and anxiety. She will learn to recognize her old patterns and habits, such as passivity, aggression, drug abuse, and sex addiction, that hindered healthy relationships. Deep relaxation and self-hypnosis may be tools she develops to help her gain control over her mind and body, relax on command, and neutralize specific fears and anxieties.

# Chapter 12

# Identity Development

I've really worked hard at not incorporating the abuse experience into my sense of self. I've been more in denial than anything else. It's too ugly to really look at very closely for any length of time. I vow that I will never treat anyone like she treated me. I am never going to be anything like her. My sisters used to say, "You're going to be just like her if you don't do this or that." That was the big threat in our family. My sister would use it, and she would say, "If you don't do this that I ask of you, you're going to be just like her then." This became the tool of manipulation in our family.

*Alana*

Perpetrators of mother-daughter incest controlled their victims methodically and repetitively by inflicting psychological trauma. Through words, they disempowered and disconnected their victims. They instilled terror and helplessness and destroyed the victims' sense of self in relation to others. The survivor fell victim to her abuser's pattern of jealous surveillance of social contacts. She was not allowed to engage in ordinary peer activities, or if she did participate her mother often intruded at will while keeping up the appearance and sustaining secrecy. Her mother induced fear through violent outbursts and chaotic, unpredictable rule enforcement. She destroyed the victim's sense of autonomy through highly organized patterns of punishment and control. She supervised what her daughter ate, when she slept, when she went to the bathroom, and what she wore. The victim was further shamed and demoralized when her mother intrusively controlled bodily functions through forced feeding, starvation, use of enemas, sleep deprivation, prolonged exposure to heat or cold, and imprisonment in closets, attics, or basements.

The mother-daughter incest survivor experienced the most severe victimization, child abuse by a close family member. She had no one to turn to for care and protection. Her traumatic experience of sexual abuse was fully incorporated into her inner world when the basic building blocks of her world as a child were still in the developmental stage. The victimization she experienced at the hands of her mother defined the world and self-assumptions of her as a developing child. As a child, she adopted negative assumptions in all domains. The trust and optimism, sense of safety and stability, the feeling of relative invincibility that are afforded the person with positively based assumptions were absent in her psychological world as an abused child. Instead, her world was largely one of anxiety, danger, and uncertainty. Her sense of self and others was powerfully affected. This total disruption may have been manifested psychologically in a basic personality disorder (Janoff-Bulman, 1992). As a child abuse victim, she perhaps displayed dysfunctions in personality and also in cognitive development. Similar to other abused children, she likely demonstrated cognitive dysfunction and also delays in age-appropriate problem-solving operations. As victims of childhood abuse, mother-daughter incest survivors are often diagnosed with learning disabilities.

Impaired identity development is a commonly reported outcome of childhood sexual abuse. For the mother-daughter incest survivor, the process of identity formation is a difficult one, a struggle and a paradox of needing to differentiate and distance herself from her mother while also yearning to connect with her mother in defining her own identity as a woman. The mother-daughter incest survivor still hoped for a meal, a bath, a comforting word, and love and acceptance while feeling overwhelmed with feelings of helplessness and confusion about who she was and what was happening to her. She became increasingly dependent on her perpetrator who continued to manipulate and control without any suspicion from the neighborhood. Her mother became a source of terror and degradation but also of comfort. She clung to her mother, to the one relationship she yearned for. This attachment became a bond of identification between the victim and perpetrator. She felt emotionally bonded to her mother; she empathized with her and saw the world through her eyes. She developed her mother's point of view and an intense worshipful adoration of her. She perceived her mother as deific, powerful, a source of strength and life itself (Karen, 1994).

The process of individuation has not produced a range of characteristics, skills, and personality traits which are uniquely her own. She may not feel grounded and secure in the world as she does not possess her own physical and mental boundaries. Being controlled and possessed by her mother has curtailed her establishment of a separate space, a unique sense of self. Repeated trauma formed and deformed her personality.

The process of separation does not establish a firm base for her to differentiate from her mother. As her boundaries were violated by her mother, she does not grow up with a clear, solid sense of self (Hyde, 1986). Through years of mother's invasion and impingement, her boundaries became unclear. She has little sense of where she begins and ends and what constitutes intrusiveness.

> My mother was so needy and controlling, so egocentric. She was totally inappropriate. Sometimes she would get so upset to the point of trying to kill me. She had no boundaries. She didn't have a very clear idea about herself. It was like I was her or something. She doesn't even know that you are a person. Neither do I.
>
> *Michelle*

Abuse at the hands of her mother has left her with a confused sense of self and a severe lack of boundaries between herself and her mother. Because her mother had poor boundaries herself, it is difficult for the survivor to learn that she has distinct boundaries. She grapples with a unique sense of self, with a separate sense of identity.

Due to the inevitable modeling relationship between mother and daughter, mother-daughter incest survivors may have impaired identification with their mothers. They were not provided with an opportunity to identify with a caregiving mother but instead experienced mothers as deficient and defective in their mothering role. Because their identity was not based on positive connectedness or a mutuality of caring, they fear themselves to be incomplete and insufficient and inadequate as mothers.

Since adolescence, the two main tasks of this developmental stage, separation and self-definition, have produced tremendous anxiety and pain for the mother-daughter incest survivor. Her adolescent experience of terror and disempowerment has effectively compromised the three normal adaptive tasks of this life stage: the formation of identity, the gradual separation from the family of origin, and the exploration of a wider social world. Identity for the mother-daughter incest survivor has not been based on positive identification, connectedness, and mutuality of caring that is found in healthy mother-daughter relationships. She has not shared empathically with her mother or maintained the well-being of their relationship. She has not developed a sense of herself as a caring being who derives strength and competence from her own relational capacities. She has not participated in mutually enhancing relationships as a child or an adult. She has no foundation of personality development.

Mother-daughter incest has a primary effect not only on psychological structures of the self but also on the systems of attachment and meaning that link individual and community. The survivor loses security, her sense of safety in the world, because her fundamental assumptions about a safe, meaningful world have been shattered. The basic foundation of trust, of faith in a world in which she could belong, was denied her. She feels completely derelict, alone, and banished from the human and divine systems that preserve life itself (Miller, 1994).

Essentially, she has been locked out of the possibilities for human connection. She feels acute loneliness which accompanies feelings of self-blame, helplessness, and powerlessness. She is left predisposed to shame and doubt, to doubt self and others. She does not feel she has the capacity to influence relationships, build empowering connections, and survive in the world. A sense of disconnection pervades every relationship. She does not experience a secure sense of connection with caring people. She has not been allowed to build her image of herself as worthy. For the rest of her life, she will struggle with self-esteem, trust, and being able to receive positive messages.

Stigmatization served to communicate negative messages to her, and these messages became integrated into her self-image. As a mother-daughter incest survivor, she received throughout her life the message that mastering her own life or becoming a worthwhile person was impossible, and that she was markedly different from other people. This contaminated, stigmatized identity became a stable part of her personality structure. As a child, a malignant sense of inner badness became the core around which her identity was formed. She persisted in her attempts to camouflage this profound sense of innate badness by placating her abuser and doing whatever was required of her to find favor in her mother's eyes. Enduring into adulthood, a perfectionist zest or forced competence may lead to substantial occupational success. Feeling inauthentic and false, she believes that if her secret and true self were uncovered, she would be shunned and berated (Rosencrans, 1997).

> It has really damaged my sense of self, my identity. I've grown up very talented musically and artistically, and I did fairly well academically and have tons of friends. I can't shake that sense of myself, though, that I have carried my mother physically and emotionally with me. It's a feeling of being so enmeshed. It's as if she is inside me and still is to quite a degree. She has this hold on me. I can't shake her, and it has affected my self-esteem and self-image. It's affected my body image to the point where I look like her, and I'd feel better if I had a different body, different from hers. My sense of achievement in the world is so tied to her. It's like whatever you do, don't do better than her. I've made sure of that in many ways.

*Mable*

The mother-daughter incest survivor may idealize and strongly attach to her mother who demonstrates a perverse fascination with her. She may perceive her father as indifferent and make attempts to preserve a bond with him. She may excuse his failure to protect her by attributing her abuse experience to her own worthlessness. She is unable to sustain glorified images of her parents as trustworthy, dependable, consistent caregivers. Unable to develop an inner sense of safety and a secure sense of independence, the mother-daughter incest survivor remains more dependent than other children on external sources of comfort and solace. She desperately and indiscriminately seeks someone to depend upon. The result is a paradox observed repeatedly in abused children; they may quickly attach to strangers but also cling to the very parent or parents who abused them (Janoff-Bulman, 1992).

The practitioner will need to be cognizant that a by-product of a neglectful environment in which chronic trauma can occur is a general loss of strength in the individual's sense of self. The mother-daughter incest survivor, who feels deficient and has difficulty defining her individuality, may give herself to others for identity and validation. She may seek nurturance and cling to intimate relationships. She may yearn for love and affection, yet still feel abandoned, hurt, and that she is still missing out. In therapy, she might wish to merge with her therapist who appears stronger and more centered. She may attempt to take on the therapist's core sense of self (Dalenberg, 2000).

> There's no question that I chose men that were very much like my mother. My sisters would point that out to me. They would say, "Wait a minute, what's going on in our collective lives anyway?" We tend to talk about this. We're very open. We've realized that our lives are not normal lives, that our lives have not been your standard run of the mill, middle-class life. We made a pact, my sisters and I, that if we ever see that we're making mistakes, that we're acting like her, that we're continuing this pattern—take out a gun and shoot us. We made a pact, an agreement, a promise to each other that if we're making mistakes, we'd point it out to one another. So we're very strong in that way. My sister visited me once and I was engaged to a fellow who was very abusive, very controlling, very nasty, and very petulant. She said, "Who does this remind you of?" I said, "Oh my god, you're right."

> *Alana*

The abuse survivor feels abandoned to her fate, and this abandonment is often resented to a greater extent than the abuse itself. In a climate of unspeakable abuse and disrupted relationships, the mother-daughter incest survivor faces the formidable developmental task of finding a way to form primary attachments to caretakers who, from her perspective, are dangerous and negligent. She must find a way to develop a sense of self in relation to others who are uncaring and cruel. She must acquire the ability to self-regulate in an environment in which her body is at the disposal of others' needs. She must find ways to self-soothe in an atmosphere without solace. In a climate that demands that she bring her will into complete conformity with that of her abuser, she must develop the capacity for initiative. She will be challenged to develop intimacy in an environment in which all intimate relationships are corrupt. She will be challenged to develop an identity out of an environment which defines her as a worthless slave. In order to preserve hope and meaning, she may reject the conclusion that something is wrong with her mother. She may go to any lengths to frame an explanation for her fate that acquits her mother of all blame and responsibility.

Because the survivor doubts herself, she may get stuck and feel unable to make choices or assert herself. She may protect herself through isolation and withdrawal. In relationships, she may feel that she is being used, that everyone wants something from her. She may always fear that the other shoe is going to fall. She may adapt to her environment of constant danger, though, by developing extraordinary abilities to alertly scan for warning signs of attack and by remaining attuned to her perpetrator's inner state. The self develops under consistent attempts to protect herself, to avert or appease her abuser, while being convinced of her utter helplessness and futility of resistance. She gains control by trying to be good while believing that her abuser has supernatural powers, can read her thoughts, and has absolute control. She may continue to struggle with her identity as a female and even reject identification with her mother's gender because she doesn't feel pride in sharing it. Over time, she may develop a more powerful image of woman, and wear femininity with greater ease.

The therapist must be aware that, due to years of isolation, alienation, oppression, suppression, and denial, it may be difficult for the mother-daughter incest survivor to find herself, to find the voice inside that is totally and honestly hers. Because she is focusing on issues of identity and intimacy, she often feels that she is in a second adolescence. She may lack social skills that typically manifest during this stage of development. She often feels awkward and self-conscious and ashamed of her backwardness in skills that other adults take for granted.

By taking inventory and getting rid of mental debris, she can make room for herself, hear her voice, find out who she is, and take possession of her life. She will need to claim her experience, to respect her thoughts and her feelings, to love and protect herself, and to believe in herself. The adult survivor will need to tell the little girl that she was hurt and victimized, that she was powerless as a child, that it was not her fault, and now the adult will take care of her and nurture her. As the trauma resides into the past, it no longer impedes intimacy. She may be ready to channel her energy more fully toward a relationship with a partner.

The trauma of mother-daughter incest calls into question basic human relationships, and breaches attachments of family, friendship, love, and community. It shatters the construction of the self that is formed and sustained in relation to others. Incest undermines the belief systems that give meaning to human experience and violates the victim's faith in a natural or divine order, thus casting the victim into a state of existential crisis (Janoff-Bulman, 1992). The mother-daughter incest survivor becomes trapped in an abusive environment and faces difficult tasks of adaptation. She is challenged to find ways to preserve a sense of trust in people who are undeserving, safety in an unsafe situation, control in an environment that can be terrifying and unpredictable, and power in a situation of monumental helplessness. Under the extreme conditions of early, severe, and prolonged abuse, she compensated through an immature system of psychological defenses, through extraordinary capacities, both creative and destructive, through severe impairments and extraordinary strengths. Her self was formed, her personality fragmented, under the burden of repeated inescapable abuse, altered states of consciousness, and a wide array of symptoms both somatic and psychological (Terr, 1994). In this pathological environment of childhood abuse, she may form separated personality fragments with separate names, functions, and memories. Fragmentation may become a defensive adaptation and the fundamental principle for her personality organization, thereby preventing the ordinary integration of knowledge, memory, emotional states, bodily experience, and identity (Waites, 1993; Cuffe and Frick-Helms, 1995).

In summary, the road to wholeness for the mother-daughter incest survivor may be a difficult one. A positive self-image has not developed. The little girl did not feel valued and respected. She could not develop autonomy or a sense of her own separation within a relationship. The trauma of her abuse experience thwarted her normal childhood development, individual competence, and capacity for initiative. The trauma robbed her of something central to who she is, something fundamental to her very being. It left her with huge feelings of guilt and inferiority. Her self-esteem was destroyed; her capacity for intimacy was compromised. In adulthood, she will be faced with the daunting task of reconstructing a self.

The critical issues in working with adult survivors of maternal incestuous abuse include the developmental process of identification and differentiation, as well as boundary formation. It is critical that the practitioner acknowledge that, given their relationships with their abusers, mother-daughter incest survivors struggle with the process of separation from their mothers. This may be one of the critical differences in this type of sexual abuse. The goal of therapy will be to suggest and encourage opportunities for identity development, self-definition, and self-regulation for the survivor so that she will be able to define herself and determine who she is apart from her mother and her incest experience. Assisting the survivor to identify her difficulty with the process of identity formation, and exploring opportunities for self-definition and self-regulation with her, encourages and promotes development of her own separate individuality. The therapist can give permission to the survivor to freely express the range of feelings toward her mother, to work through her fears of being like her mother, and to see herself differently from her mother. Ultimately, she can be assisted to reintegrate into her own identity those healthy, nonabusive parts of her mother.

# Chapter 13

# Parenting

I've always wanted to be around kids and to teach them, but I have very ambivalent feelings because I think I am a monster who could destroy. I have an impulse to abuse a child, so I cut children out of my life completely. Part of my fear is that it'll bring up my own experience. It relates to my doubt and fear that I could perpetrate.

*Alice*

Adult survivors of childhood sexual abuse worry about their own parenting skills. Some are afraid of becoming parents themselves because they believe they would be inadequate parents. Many are concerned about the intergenerational implications of abuse, and that they may victimize their own children. Some survivors feel so terrible about themselves that they are reluctant to have children because the children may be like them. Some strive to become better parents than the parents they had as children.

Mother-daughter incest survivors have these fears intensified. They are left with considerable confusion regarding their own identities as women, and with tremendous fear and doubt regarding their own competence as mothers.

I actually thought of giving up my first two kids. They're two years apart. They felt too perfect, and I was afraid I was just going to ruin them. I felt even if I just touched them I was going to poison them.

*Michelle*

They report profound fear and anxiety about being like their mothers. They may be reluctant to disclose their abuse experience because they fear that people will undoubtedly classify them as damaged, reprehensible, and unfit as women and mothers. They fear that people will think they, too, are perpetrators of child sexual abuse. Due to the unhealthy role modeling from her sexually abusive mother, the adult survivor of maternal incestuous abuse has tremendous fear that she will abuse her own children.

> My biggest fear about having children is not that I would sexually or physically abuse them, but that I would emotionally abuse because I would be so needy that I would end up abusing. I want to have children, but I'd never want to do that to them. I wouldn't want to be responsible for that. I think I would kill myself if I ever thought I was going to hurt a child. I don't want anybody to go through what I had to go through.
>
> *Sonia*

> I'm afraid I'd be neglectful and that I wouldn't have good boundaries. I have a lot of fears around that I'd be emotionally unavailable more than anything and that I couldn't take care of them.
>
> *Mable*

The clinician must be open to the possibility that mother-daughter incest survivors, who are themselves mothers, may present with deep concern and intense fear about continuing the cycle of abuse. For those women who are aware that their mothers had been sexually abused in childhood, their concerns that sexual abuse is somehow passed on through families is exacerbated. The fear of becoming an abuser may result in her distancing herself from her children, especially her daughters.

> I had such fear about being a mother myself. With my own children, I was very careful around their caretaking, changing them and bathing them. When they were old enough, I'd let them clean themselves or I'd ask my husband to do personal care for them if I didn't feel that it was appropriate for me. I consciously

made the decision to break the cycle of abuse. I encourage privacy and I don't enter the bathroom when they are in there. I always knock on the door before I enter their rooms.

*Ashley*

Many mother-daughter incest survivors choose to not have children at all. Many often believe they should have been aborted by their mother, so why should they have children. For many of those women, this fear results in seeking counseling services to assist them with the establishment and maintenance of physical and psychological boundaries. As parents, they may be inconsistent, rigid, or too permissive. They may believe that their sexually abusive mother poisoned their potential to become healthy mothers themselves.

When mother-daughter incest survivors become parents, they often do not want their mother near the babies. Some even deny access to the mother-in-law due to deep fears and anxiety about having any woman near their children. Some mothers lack trust and experience anxiety about bathing their children since their mother abused them frequently at bath times. For many mothers who overprotect their children, learning to trust is a huge challenge.

Finally, many survivors who are mothers report experiencing difficulty in their mothering role, particularly in terms of establishing appropriate boundaries with their children. Some mothers who find themselves crossing the line with their children, physically, emotionally, and/or sexually, ideally will enter therapy to deal with this issue. It is imperative that the therapist discuss the limits of confidentiality with the client. The therapist must be able to ask the mother-daughter incest survivor if she has offended because the survivor may be playing out her own sexual abuse with another child. Mother-daughter incest survivors may need assistance in learning about the parameters of healthy parent-child relationships and in setting realistic expectations for themselves regarding their maternal role. Teaching parenting skills may be an essential component of the counseling process.

# Chapter 14

# Treating the Adult Victim

I do feel compassion for her and if I were to express it to her I'd be open for more abuse. I still am open for more abuse if I talk to her. She wants everything to be normal. Once when I was setting boundaries with her she broke down sobbing. I didn't know what to do and that angered me because once again I was taking care of her. She ropes me in. I always talk about the hook. It's a push and a pull and so confusing.

*Lisa*

The personality that is formed in an atmosphere of coercive control is not well adapted to adult life. Survivors of childhood abuse are left with fundamental problems in basic trust, autonomy, and initiative. They approach the tasks of early adulthood, establishing independence and intimacy, burdened by major impairments in self-care, in cognition and memory, in identity, and in the capacity to form stable relationships. Their intimate relationships are driven by the hunger for protection and care and are haunted by the fear of abandonment or exploitation, of domination and betrayal. Repeated abuse is not actively sought but rather passively encountered as an unavoidable dreadful fate, accepted as the inevitable price of relationships (van Wormer, 2001). The child victim, now grown, seems fated to relive her traumatic experiences not only in memory but also in daily life. It is not uncommon, then, to find adult survivors who continue to minister to the wishes and needs of those who once victimized them and who continue to permit major intrusions without boundaries or limits. It is not uncommon for the survivor of childhood abuse to experience such profound deficiency in self-protection or self-agency that the notion of having choice, or saying no to the emotional demands of a parent, spouse, lover, or authority figure is completely inconceivable.

Adult survivors of mother-daughter incest often feel like mindless objects still under mother's total control. This dynamic often sets them up for continued attacks on their mind and body. Part of this dynamic involves an attitude on the part of the adult victim that she lives with implications of abuse every day, that it's current, real, and not in the past. Part of this dynamic stems from her abusive childhood in which she may have been intensely attached to and protective of her abusive mother. Connection to her abusive mother may have been her emotional lifeline. In her childhood environment of violation, betrayal, and pain, she also received food, shelter, and perhaps some nurturing. Even the pain and fear associated with the trauma of her abuse may become transformed into her feeling connected to her mother. Whether she was being beaten or violated and afterward cuddled and caressed, constantly touched by her hypersolicitous caretaker, or scolded by her neglectful mother, she at the same time may have felt appreciated and needed. She may have grown up thinking pain was synonymous with connectedness. She may have felt special, chosen, and singled out for this sort of connection. This may set the stage, then, for the adult victim's continued involvement in a similar relationship with her mother, since in her mind it may be the only way to achieve and maintain this connection, to satisfy her longing for maternal love and approval.

> I think I was attempting to please her in many respects. Of course you always hope right until the end that there's going to be some reconciliation, some resolution. I believe in miracles. I believe that it's wonderful being human because we have the capacity to change, regardless of what's gone before. You always hope that in your own family and in your own life the potential for that exists.
>
> *Alana*

Adult victims of mother-daughter incest, perhaps more than other abuse victims, may feel tremendous frustration about not being able to take control over themselves. They fear that they will never escape their mothers' legacies. They may have been violated for so long by their mothers that they got used to it. Adult victims of maternal incestuous abuse have been robbed of any positive feelings they have about themselves. It is easy for them to believe hurtful words, to feel self-contempt and a lack of faith in self. They may struggle with the whole notion of recovery, of being a survivor, when they feel like human refuse.

Mother-daughter incest survivors may want to separate and disown their mothers, but the fear of being judged when they vocalize this keeps the survivors tied to their mothers. It contributes to the feelings of betrayal, isolation, guilt, and stigmatization they feel as a result of their abuse experience. Adult victims may, in spite of their abuse experience, feel incredible loyalty to their mothers and guilt about not trying hard enough to forgive them. Many feel that there is something wrong with them, that it is their fault, if they do not forgive their abusers. Some feel disloyal when they talk to anyone about the issues. Many find themselves nursing their abusers in illness, defending their abusers in adversity, and even continuing to submit to their sexual demands.

Many adult survivors may choose not to talk about their abusive past so as to maintain a relationship and a pretense that their mother-daughter relationship is normal. The perpetrator may have convinced her daughter to resist disclosure of their little secret. This secret may continue as a companion for the adult victim, similar to a friend, or a child she owns and keeps hidden away. She may keep the secret of her childhood abusive experience as a vital aspect of feeling she is in control of her life. This secret may become a substitute, however, for relationships with other people. It may reinforce her experience of guilt and profound isolation. It may serve to "shame trap" her so that she feels ashamed of her needs, ashamed of her relationship with her mother, and stuck in a self-generated feedback loop of more shame and abuse. Caught up in the "worthlessness cycle," her fear keeps her locked in a pattern of shame and abuse at the hands of her mother (Bepko and Krestan, 1990). This pattern may escalate to the extent that she perceives herself as bad and becomes convinced that others will sense her innate badness if they get too close.

For those adult women who remain close to their abusive mothers, confusion, lack of boundaries, and inappropriate behaviors may continue on the part of the mother. Many grown daughters feel compelled to maintain or reestablish a relationship with their mothers. Societal expectations and social pressures to remain close to the mother make it difficult for these women to disconnect. Social pressure to maintain a relationship with the mother may result in suppression of anger and hostility toward the mother. Clinicians will need to support these daughters as they cope with conflicting feelings about remaining in contact with Mom or disengaging from her.

> It is really complicated for me. There are times I want to love her so much, and there are other times I just want to put a hatchet to her heart. I'm not sure what to do.
>
> *Page*

The adult victim of maternal incestuous abuse may crave a relationship with her mother. She may not reconcile herself to the notion that she will not have a healthy relationship with her mother. She may go on dreaming, hoping, and wishing that her mother will one day love and nurture her. A mother's touch may be desperately desired and actually sought by the daughter. Her need for human connection, to feel safe and cared for, may set the stage for toleration of her mother's touch. Many adult survivors will feel emotionally and/or physically frozen, or numbed when touched by their mothers. This feeling of immobilization may occur in a variety of situations and may trigger unpleasant memories, flashbacks, or panic attacks.

Many daughters will carry these feelings of being immobilized, of being flooded with too many emotions, into their relationships, in particular, relationships with their daughters. They may feel tremendous sadness and shame about the discomfort they feel with their own daughters. They may share this discomfort with their mothers, and take a risk by communicating to their mothers about their abuse. Many choose to keep quiet, however, because they anticipate that their mothers will deny the sexual abuse, attack them for causing such a disturbance, and turn other family members against them. Many daughters believe that confronting their mothers and exploring the past will lead to greater problems. Hence, they make the decision to carry the secret, to remain silent in order to maintain peace in the family, and maintain some kind of relationship with their mother. Many daughters will do almost anything to believe that they are loved like other children by their mothers (Rosencrans, 1997).

The literature identifies the incestuous mother as relying on the daughter for love and mothering, attention, affection, and emotional support (McCarthy, 1986; Ogilvie, 1996). Mother-daughter incest survivors experience their mothers as lonely, in need of intimacy, dependent, isolated, insecure, inadequate, unstable, and unempathic. Even in adulthood, mother-daughter incest survivors often struggle to, as one survivor explained, "avoid the lasso or fish line, and loosen their mothers' grip on them." Many daughters may end or greatly restrict their relationship with their mothers in order for them to move forward in their lives. Ultimately, it may be left to the daughter to determine how much separation or distance to take. Because these mothers may resent or resist any individuation by their daughters, they may try to manipulate or control their daughters so they will remain enmeshed.

Mother-daughter incest survivors, who may continue to be victimized in adulthood by their mothers, will need assistance in negotiating their present relationships with their mothers. It may be difficult for the adult survivor to emerge from her cocoon and begin her transformation if she continues to be victimized as an adult by her mother. She will need to set more appropriate physical and psychological boundaries between herself and her mother. She may need coaching in the area of boundary formation as well as support as she copes with conflicting feelings regarding closeness and separation. She may find moving away and distancing herself from her mother a very difficult task to complete.

> I feel a horrible amount of sadness about not being able to rescue her, not being able to save her and to stop the abuse. I eventually got to the point where I realized that I wasn't responsible for the way she turned out, the person she ended up becoming. We all have to take a sense of accountability for our lives. But I remember being really unhappy about the fact that I couldn't love her enough to save her from herself. There was no escape from it. I could walk away from her, and I did, but she remained that person until the end of her life. She never had a sense of real happiness. Despite all that, I did love her.
>
> *Alana*

The mother-daughter incest survivor, like other oppressed people, believes that she has limited options in life and that rejection is the norm. She continues to live in terror that life is going to deal her a huge blow, that tragedy is inevitable. Feelings of powerlessness and worthlessness exacerbate feelings of frustration about not being able to master her life. This mind-set may set the stage for further victimization by her mother.

> She paved the way for me to be further victimized, violated by others. Without question, I've picked out situations where I've done that to myself. I have to acknowledge that part of overcoming this is refusing to be a victim. I have to accept responsibility for my choices. No one has a gun to my head. No one makes me get into these relationships. I've chosen them. There's big posters on the road that say, "Don't go here," the old saying about going down a road and you fall into a pit. Well, the first time you didn't know it was there, and the second time, you know that this pit is in the road. If you're going down that road, you made that choice. I think by taking responsibility for it, you sort of start monitoring yourself. You do a little bit of self-talk internally and say, "Uh-uh, you're not going to do this to me; you're not going to get away with this."

*Alana*

The clinician will need to understand that many mother-daughter incest survivors live in an environment of totalitarian control, often executed by violent means and death threats, arbitrary enforcement of petty rules, periodic rewards, and destruction of rival relationships through isolation, secrecy, and betrayal (Davies and Frawley, 1994). Mother-daughter incest survivors develop under these conditions of domination and control and pathological attachments to those who abuse and neglect them. They may strive to maintain these attachments even if it means sacrificing their own welfare, their own reality, and their own lives (Briere, 1996). They may look outside of themselves, even to their abusive mothers, to confirm that they are worth something, to give them affirmation.

> For a long time, I would be doing things and seeking her approval. I would still want to hear her tell me that it was okay and that I had done a great job. Even now to this day, I still want her approval.

*Iris*

The therapist must realize that it may take a long period of time for the adult victim to accept that she has a right to her anger, that she has the right to disengage from her mother in order to move on with her life. While understanding that the daughter may struggle with individuation, the clinician will need to be aware that she may also have difficulty being alone. The clinician can help nurture a more positive, trusting attitude in the client. Over time, the client will come to trust her own ability to discern what is good and not good for her. She needs to believe in her own self-control and self-mastery and that she can do what is best for her. She will need to be encouraged to learn how to give to herself, to look after her needs, and to incorporate into her life people and activities that make her feel good about herself. She will need to distance herself from those who disbelieve and from those who hurt and diminish her.

> There was a lot of self-doubt and self-incrimination. I think if you're going through this, just be patient. Love yourself. Be accepting of yourself. Allow yourself to see it for what it is. Don't be a victim. Life is more than a few years of your life. Life is out there; it's in front of you. It's not behind you. It's not in the past. That's not where your life is. That part is over. It's finished. That person can't hurt you anymore. Just draw some strength from that and realize that it's okay to go forward. It's all right. You have to go forward. There is no other choice.
>
> *Alana*

A full exploration of the possible consequences of severing or attempting to repair the daughter's relationship with her mother is a necessary prerequisite to any therapeutic action involving the abuser. If the mother-daughter relationship is so fractured that no healthy aspects of the relationship can be identified by the client, the counselor may assist in identifying other adult women who can symbolically serve the function of female role model.

If she chooses to confront her mother about her abuse, it is essential that she anticipate rejection, or that her mother may minimize what she tells her. She also needs to know that her mother may not show remorse, apologize, or admit to her perpetration. Instead, she may be defensive and angry. With her therapist, the mother-daughter incest survivor can rehearse and role-play the confrontation, and explore what she needs for herself. The clinician must acknowledge that the client can stand up for herself as a powerful adult, that she can end the silence surrounding her abuse, and cease protecting the abuser. The clinician will need to support the client if she decides to take her power back without directly confronting her mother but rather through role-playing and letter writing. The mother-daughter incest survivor needs to be encouraged to keep talking to people she trusts, read books, keep a journal, join a group, continue in therapy, and trust herself. She will need to tap into those resources that are available to her and to access her personal strengths and courage. She needs to understand that healing will come with loving relationships, acknowledging that she is a good person, and appreciating who she is.

> My self-esteem still waivers quite a bit, but the constant rein-
> forcement I get from my relationships with my colleagues, my
> husband, and my children leaves me feeling that I am a good
> person.
>
> *Ashley*

> I suffered through periods of depression, through severe feel-
> ings of inferiority. Even in a business environment when I was
> excelling, I was constantly second-guessing my own progress.
> It was never good enough. But this doesn't have to ruin a per-
> son's life. You can come through it. You can achieve a lot of joy
> and happiness in your life. You can have good relationships. It's
> a lot of hard work, and it takes time. It's taken me twenty-odd
> years. I certainly wasn't always this centered and confident and
> happy.
>
> *Alana*

Whatever the client decides to do about confronting her mother, it is important that it feels right for her, that it meets her expectations of her own needs. Through group therapy, the mother-daughter survivor can receive support from group members and can take the opportunity to share her feelings and concerns regarding experiences with her mother. She may choose to remain close to her mother. Open relationships with supportive family members may be sought. She may empower herself to take breaks from her family, in particular her mother, for months, even years. She may choose to discuss her mother's childhood with her, to gain understanding and put her own experience in context. She may discover that her mother is an abuse survivor herself, which may assist her efforts toward reconciliation with her mother and other family members.

> As an adult, I do understand that there are certain patterns there. She was abused sexually, physically, and emotionally. She grew up in a very constrictive family situation. My grandmother, a staunch Catholic, looked the other way at pedophile activities of my grandfather. My mom definitely grew up in an insane environment. She simply didn't break free from it. She couldn't break the pattern. She continued it to a large extent. There was a lot of coercion in the family. She was a very coercive individual. I saw her as having a very limited existence, a very failed existence. One of the keystones of my life is that perhaps her life will not be in vain if mine isn't. If I can make my life count, if I can do things in an environmental context to make the world a better place, if I can inspire people that I meet, if I can be loving, good and kind, then perhaps it wasn't all for nothing. I'm a product of her. Whether I'd like to embrace that or not, I am. I'm very grateful for her for without her, I wouldn't be here. I wouldn't be breathing. I love my life and I'm very glad that I have a shot at it, that I have the possibilities that I have. If it were not for her genetic input, at the very least, I would not be here. So I can't malign her too much because I am really grateful for what she has given me. She's given me life, and I'm glad about that.

> *Alana*

In summary, the survivor often finds herself entangled in a complicated relationship with her abuser. She may enter therapy because of ongoing conflict in her relationship with her mother. Often some degree of coercive control may still be present in the relationship with her mother, and occasionally the sexual abuse itself is still occurring. The clinician should never assume that the sexual abuse stopped in childhood. He or she will need to carefully explore the particulars of the survivor's present relationship with her mother. If she chooses to resume or maintain contact with her mother, it is vitally important that she set the ground rules in order to feel safe and in charge of herself. The clinician will need to help the client set boundaries and to take better care of herself so that she can define what contact, if any, she wishes to maintain with her mother. She will need to give herself permission to leave her mother when the relationship feels abusive or when her needs are not being met. She can ask for an apology from her mother and even ask her to enter therapy. Her mother's control over her will diminish as a result of her defining and setting the limits of the relationship.

> I still feel some responsibility for my mother, but she is not willing to seek help. I still love her, but I know a relationship is not possible unless she seeks help. I have asked her, but I know that it is highly unlikely that she will seek help.

*Ashley*

# PART V:
# SPECIAL ISSUES

In addition to Part IV, which addresses counseling issues unique to the phenomenon of mother-daughter incest, this section of the book draws specific attention to the following topics of particular importance to the therapist working with mother-daughter incest survivors:

1. Stepmother versus biological mothers
2. Therapist gender
3. Transference
4. Countertransference

In keeping with the previous sections of the book, counseling strategies and treatment suggestions are made to assist practitioners with these issues.

# Chapter 15

# Stepmothers versus Biological Mothers

What about the mother-child bond? Where the hell was mine?
Why didn't she bond with me . . . comfort me . . . hold me and
chase away all the boogiemen and kiss all of my booboos
better?

*Taylore*

Sexual abuse of a child by a more powerful adult has a traumatic
impact on the life of the victim. When the adult is a family friend, as
is often the case, somehow as a society it is easier for us to swallow or
to understand in a way. When the abuse is incestuous, the scars from
the victimization are deep and long lasting.

Sexual abuse by a female, particularly in a mothering role, is more
difficult to understand due to cultural images of motherhood. "A
mother is a life force, a spirit. She is living, loving energy, channeling
into all our lives. A mother's experience extends far beyond her own
offspring. She is a universal person; her strength comes gently"
(Weber, as cited in Lanese, 1998, p. 32). "There is no other closeness
in human life like the closeness between a mother and her child.
Chronologically, physically and spiritually, they are just a few heart-
beats away from being the same person" (Cheever, as cited in Lanese,
1998, p. 31). One cannot downplay the significance of the mother-
daughter bond and how it relates to personal and cultural denial of the
existence of mother-daughter incest.

Sexual abuse by a stepmother has a devastating effect on the lives
of its victims. From the victim's point of view, sexual abuse by her
stepmother represents a physical and psychological violation. It is
not uncommon for the stepdaughter to report that abuse at the hands
of her stepmother translated into an experience that is reprehensible,
that sets her apart from other human beings and leaves her feeling dif-

ferent from everyone else, hollowed out and deeply ashamed. As a child, she was not provided for. She felt unnurtured and unsafe in her family. The only mother she knew, the one person who was supposed to look after her, committed the ultimate betrayal, the most profound disconnection possible in her world.

For survivors of biological mother-perpetrated abuse, the relationship with the mother is best characterized by the most severe physical, psychological, and spiritual disconnections. These women feel deceived, deserted, betrayed, confused, offended, and intruded upon to the very core of their existence. If their biological mother, who conceived them, carried them, and delivered them, a woman of the same sex, who was once a little girl herself, victimizes them, deceives them, and rejects them, then the victims are left feeling alien-like, less than human, damaged, and unbelievably tainted. They carry with them confusion about who they are, and they struggle to make sense of this atrocity. Essentially, they maneuver as best they can in a world that isolates, disbelieves, and ignores them.

Abuse at the hands of a biological mother may be more shameful and stigmatizing for the victim given societal expectations and definitions regarding motherhood and the strength and importance of the mother-daughter dyad. Victims consistently describe a profound betrayal of trust because the perpetrator was their mother thus contributing to the high degree of traumatization for the victims. "From society's point of view, no one else can take a mother's place. No tie in life is as strong or lasting as that of a child to her mother" (Weber, as cited in Lanese, 1998, p. 32).

The most difficult issue in the survivor's life is the fact that as a child she was abused by her own mother. She describes the impact of the abuse as so devastating that not only has it affected the rest of her life, but it was "psychologically indigestible" (Evert and Bijkerk, 1987). To actually begin to live with the awareness that her own mother used her for sexual purposes is the most devastating experience she has had to endure. As a child she naturally called out for the comfort of her mother, who at the same time incomprehensibly posed the gravest threat to her well-being.

> I think, if my mother didn't want me, why didn't she give me up? I wish she would have dropped me off. I hope she's living in so much pain, because I've never lived. I hope her life is full of hell because mine has been. If this is love, I want hate.

My mother knew what she was doing to me. It was right out front; nothing was hidden. If I wasn't doing any sexual things with her, I wasn't allowed home. A lot of people tell me, if I had a childhood like yours, I would have committed suicide. I think I have died inside emotionally. I don't have emotions like you do. I don't understand why today I want to be part of your world.

*Moe*

It may be more threatening for victims to acknowledge or admit that their biological mothers abused them. It appears that more shame and stigma occurs if victims have been abused by their biological mothers. To these victims, the biological bond between them and their mothers makes the abuse more difficult to accept and disclosure more difficult. In their minds, if their perpetrator was a stepmother, then the mothering role is different. The unique tie between mother and daughter is missing. The bond between both parties is unlike that of a biological tie, a lifeline held taut between mothers and daughters which begins with the umbilical connection.

Whether the perpetrator is a stepmother or a biological mother, mother-daughter incest victims receive little nurturance and guidance from their mothers when they are growing up. They express anguish and dejection over the absence of a trusted figure. They often ventilate feelings of extreme hostility and anger as a result of feeling cheated of the kind of relationship they deserved with their mothers. They report confusion, anger, and a profound sense of loss about the fact that their mothers did not bond with them. It is critical that the practitioner be cognizant that due to cultural images of mother as protector and nurturer, survivors of mother-daughter incest reportedly experience deep wounding which leaves a devastating effect on their lives. Counseling interventions will ideally focus on identity development as well as help the survivor to cope with issues of profound betrayal, abandonment, deep-rooted shame, and self-blame.

# Chapter 16

# Therapist Gender

Researchers and practitioners continue to stress the importance of the therapeutic alliance between client and therapist. Individual therapy is a private relationship, and the role of the therapist is significant during the therapeutic process. Kaplan (1991) emphasized that gender is a significant variable in building human relationships, and that the sexes differ psychologically in their moral reasoning, modes of communication, definitions and experiences of success, and possibly the course of psychological development. This has real implications to the issue of client and therapist match, and to the effectiveness of the therapeutic process.

A mother-daughter incest survivor may experience her therapist as extremely helpful, no help at all, or even damaging. She first and foremost seeks counseling services from a listening, supportive adult who can be trusted. The mother-daughter incest survivor strives to connect with a sensitive, caring therapist who encourages her to show her real self, to express feelings, and let the pain out. She hopes her therapist is knowledgeable about sexual abuse, and more important, about the salient issues regarding mother-daughter incest. She hopes that her therapist will be open to addressing gender issues, power imbalances, and sexual violence (Bilker, 1993).

A mother-daughter incest survivor may choose a female therapist because she may believe that a woman better understands what it is like to be female, a mother, a daughter. The female practitioner may be more familiar with the dynamics of the mother-daughter dyad. She may have a better grasp of the client's pain because of her own identity issues, and issues of separation and differentiation from mother. Female therapists may have a greater awareness of the issue of body awareness, and firsthand understanding of the emotional, physical, sexual, and spiritual experiences of being female. They may have

personal and professional experience with contemporary role conflicts for females in our society.

Unique dynamics may develop when the helping relationship is
with a female. The mother-daughter incest survivor might search for
a "mothering" therapist to nurture her and protect her since she was
denied this as a child. At the other extreme, the mother-daughter incest survivor may struggle with trusting a female. She may fear that
she will be violated and abandoned once again by a woman. She may
instead gravitate toward a male therapist because she believes she
would be safe and protected in the relationship. She may base her
preference on the belief that she cannot trust a female therapist. She
may, on the other hand, choose a female therapist because her father
was emotionally and physically absent in her childhood and was not
there for her to turn to for protection. Perhaps he turned a blind eye to
the abuse that was happening at the hands of her mother.

When exploring the issue of who can best serve the mother-daughter incest survivor, a male or a female therapist, the following questions demand attention:

1. Who can best understand the life experience of a woman?
2. Who can sit with the mother-daughter incest survivor as she expresses residual rage about her childhood, tremendous feelings
   of grief and loss and betrayal?
3. Who will sustain connection with the mother-daughter incest
   survivor when she feels alone with her feelings and when she
   works through painful memories of abuse at the hands of her
   mother?
4. Who will maintain connection with the mother and survivor
   when treatment continues for a long duration?
5. Who can understand the power that a mother has over a daughter?
6. Who understands the importance of not judging, dismissing,
   dominating, or distancing?

Dealing with the mother-daughter incest survivor's issues requires
a great deal of patience, persistence, and courage for any therapist,
male or female. No consistent evidence indicates that a particular
client-therapist gender match is most effective for working with
mother-daughter incest survivors. Awareness on the part of both the

client and the therapist of the pitfalls and advantages of male and female practitioners may help make the course of therapy less bumpy.

Whether male or female, the practitioner must express a sensitivity to the client's pain and to issues regarding separation and identification with her mother. Clearly, the helping professional (male or female) must be cognizant that the mother-daughter incest survivor may have difficulty labeling her abuse or in revealing that her mother sexually abused her. The practitioner needs to acknowledge that the mother-daughter incest survivor may fear that she will frighten her therapist away. She may be wary of closeness to a female therapist and may feel threatened by her based on fears of homosexuality.

A mother-daughter incest survivor may fear identification with a female therapist because she sees a resemblance to her mother. This may result in her decision to originally choose a male therapist, or to withdraw from the female therapist once she is in the process of therapy. The client may view her female therapist as a superwoman causing her to feel angry or to be anxious about becoming overdependent. Mother-daughter incest survivors may feel a regressive pull toward their mothers and have ambivalent feelings about emotional and physical closeness to females in general. Such individuals may fare better by developing a trusting relationship with a male practitioner.

The female practitioner will need to guard against her countertransference problems with separation from the client and her tendencies toward overprotection of the client. She may be more susceptible to countertransference issues concerning pain avoidance. She may be at a higher risk or have expectations to be overly maternal and nurturing. She will need to exercise caution lest the client become too dependent, leaving the therapist drained, angry, and distant (Bilker, 1993). She will need to guard against wanting to withdraw from the client or bolt into self-protection, thereby hindering success in therapy.

> Once I disclosed to my therapist about my mother, she three weeks later announced that she was going to terminate me. I'm sure it's because she had tons of stuff around the incest as the therapist is a mother of three, one of them a baby. I'm sure I pushed all her buttons although she wasn't sexually abused herself. Stuff around being a good mother and guilt is huge. I'm sure that was it. That gave me the message that it wasn't okay to disclose, and this can happen when you tell people about the ug-

liness of being abused by your mother. I started really flipping out, so I had to quickly find a therapist who could deal with mother issues. Even though my present therapist has not been sexually abused by her mother, she was certainly physically abused. She has had to work through similar issues and is allowing me to go to that place. I really started letting it out with her physically, emotionally, and integrating it with body work.

*Mable*

The practitioner must recognize that the issue of therapist gender is an important one; in the case of mother-daughter incest, it requires particular attention given the nature of the abuse experience of mother-daughter incest survivors. Relationship dynamics may occur when a mother-daughter incest survivor chooses a male counselor.

I'm not at all comfortable with a male therapist. There always seems to be a sexual overtone for me. I don't know where I stand. Maybe that is a result of being sexually abused. I don't know what is expected of me with a male therapist. Somehow I feel that I should be sexual somehow, that it is expected of me. He's a man and I am a woman, so I have to be sexual one way or another. I must have a sexual role here, so even that's not comfortable for me.

*Sonia*

When the mother-daughter incest survivor chooses a male therapist, she may be basing her preference on the belief that she cannot trust a female therapist. Many female practitioners work with maternal abuse survivors, and it is therefore critical that they familiarize themselves with the unique dynamics which may develop when the counselor is female.

The therapist will need to maintain connection with the mother-daughter incest survivor particularly when she works through painful memories of victimization and betrayal. The client may need help as she finds positive memories about her childhood and as she integrates positive experiences of her mother into her identity. The goal in therapy will be to help the client manage her life, discuss in therapy about how normal her responses are to abnormal events, and find ways of coping with the knowledge that she was sexually abused at the hands of her mother. The goal of the therapist is to support the mother-daughter incest survivor throughout the process so that she can move beyond it. The better supported the survivor, the quicker the recovery.

> What worked for me in therapy was having a really straightforward therapist. I went to see him because I had a stillborn son and I had issues remaining from that. I became bulimic for a short period of time. Once again, I had control issues. I was not your garden variety bulimic in that I was able to very simply tell myself that I wasn't going to do this to myself anymore. Many bulimics need ongoing psychiatric care but that wasn't necessary for me and it was a very short period of time. Therapy gave me an opportunity to ask a lot of hard questions about myself and my relationship with my mother and my childhood issues. He really validated for me that I was one of the most normal, one of the sanest and most well-balanced individuals he had come across. I had spent so much time in introspection that it made me feel really good to have that experience that I was okay.
>
> *Alana*

# Chapter 17

# Transference

The process of transference refers to the client's unconscious and inappropriate perceptions and expectations of others, including therapists, based upon prior life experiences (Briere, 1989). The client, by entering therapy seeking help and care, voluntarily submits to an unequal relationship in which the therapist has superior status and power. Transference in the therapeutic process exists when clients relate to practitioners as if they were some other significant figure in their lives. Transferential feelings related to their childhood experience of dependence on their parents are inevitably stirred, further embellish the power imbalance in the therapeutic relationship, and render them vulnerable to exploitation (van Wormer, 2001).

Transference is likely to be unavoidable for the mother-daughter incest survivor. The mother-daughter incest survivor may relate to other people in her life as if they were members of her childhood family. Difficulty arises when she is unable to keep her current relationships separate from unresolved feelings toward members of her family. Transferred feelings may lead her to acting-out behaviors during therapy, which may include a variety of reactions toward the therapist. To the mother-daughter incest survivor, her counselor may seem like her dad or her mom. She may feel anger toward the world for not acknowledging the existence of the phenomenon of mother-daughter incest. In general, she may feel resentful, betrayed, and ripped off by anyone who crosses her path.

Helping professionals should not be surprised when clients direct feelings to them that are really meant for other figures in their lives, notably members of their childhood families. It is crucial in the therapeutic process that the therapist resist the temptation to abandon the client or terminate therapy. Such emotional abandonment would only replicate the original parental disconnection with the child. The clinician must deliver the message that he or she is willing to bear the unbearable, tolerate, contain, and process the information that is shared about the profound neglect and abuse suffered by the client as a child.

The mother-daughter incest survivor may feel exploited by her therapist and respond with tremendous defensiveness. She may mistrust, doubt, and become suspicious of her therapist. She may assume that her therapist cannot bear to hear the details of her traumatic abuse experience or that she is unable or unwilling to help. She may feel intimidated by her therapist, as she did by her parents, as someone who is in a position of authority.

The therapist may be seen by the mother-daughter incest survivor as the "good parent" or the "bad parent," paralleling her childhood dynamic to love or hate her parent(s). She may hope that her therapist will meet her intense need for love and nurturance. The greater the mother-daughter incest survivor's emotional contention of helplessness and abandonment, the more likely she is to cast the therapist in the role of omnipotent rescuer. In her perception of the therapist as an authority figure, a parent, or as someone who is very nurturing, she may feel attracted to her therapist and sexually fantasize about him or her. She may insist on a sexual relationship as the only convincing gesture of the therapist's caring and commitment. She may immediately expect her female therapist to look after her, protect her, and be her caregiver. When these idealized expectations are not met, she may feel betrayed, rejected, hurt, angered, and even neglected or abused by her therapist. She may express immense rage toward the therapist as a result of displaced anger toward her mother. The reverse may take place as well when confronted or angered by the therapist.

The mother-daughter incest survivor may repress or deny her feelings for a variety of reasons. Perhaps as a child, she was to be "seen and not heard" and, as an adult, she may find it easy or natural to behave in a similar fashion. Some of what is happening to her in her life may be distorted in fact to fit in with old abusive family patterns or belief systems.

> This projective identification may lead the client to scrutinize every word and gesture from the therapist. It may also draw the therapist into unaccustomed hostile reactions, and into dynamics of dominance and submission, thereby inadvertently reenacting aspects of the abusive relationship at the hands of her mother. (Herman, 1992, p. 140)

Projection may play a part as innocent actions by the therapist are transformed into acts of cruelty by their symbolic value for the traumatized client. The mother-daughter incest survivor may seek to find an enemy on whom to vent her rage at the unfairness of life. Identification with her parent perpetrator can lead her to abusively penetrate the therapist's boundaries, making entitled demands for time and attention (Dalenberg, 2000).

The mother-daughter incest survivor may use anger as an attachment strategy, particularly if she feels an insecure attachment to her therapist and/or others in her life. Such anger is likely to surface when she is under great distress and feeling insecure and anxious about abandonment. Anxiety and anger are natural strategies used by the mother-daughter incest survivor to protest the disappearance or temporary unavailability of an attachment figure. She may respond in an exaggerated manner to the therapist's mild anger or annoyance. She may become disabled by anxiety or disengage, dissociate, or shut down. Her struggle with dependency on her therapist, which frequently occurs with trauma clients who fear trusting a powerful figure, often leads her to fear termination of therapy. She may report fearing regression after termination and profound anxiety over losing the most meaningful relationship she has ever had (Bowlby, 1988).

Practitioners will need to be sensitive to subtle cues of anger and to seek clarification from the mother-daughter incest survivor concerning what seems abusive to her. Therapists must be open to assisting the mother-daughter incest survivor with identification of anger and other feelings. The client can be encouraged to appropriately direct feelings, to gain insight into the roots of her anger and how she displaces it. She can gain understanding in terms of how feelings, fears, defenses, and reactions, both positive and negative, are projected onto significant others in her life. She can recognize the power she has as an adult, that she has control over her feelings without projecting anger and rage at significant others in her life, including the therapist.

It is important for the practitioner to understand that building attachments to those who had insecure attachments to their parents is an arduous process. The mother-daughter incest survivor may experience her or him as an unseeing, neglectful, uninvolved parent. She may view the therapist as a hostile parent who neglected to care for her and may choose to lash out at the therapist. When the mother-daughter incest survivor feels crazy, frightened, disorganized, and out of control, her transference may fluctuate between an increased need to connect with the therapist and increased mistrust, resulting in a desire to disconnect or get away from the therapist. She yearns for and simultaneously fears an adult figure who might set appropriate boundaries. She may sabotage her progress or smash hope in order to maintain control or to stave off what she perceives might be an inevitable disappointment.

She may mistrust her therapist's motives and misinterpret his or her reactions, especially when the therapist does not back away. She often accuses her therapist of exploitative or voyeuristic motives, fearing further victimization, yet she seems unable to protect herself, and reenacts the dynamics of dominance and submission. She may be frightened or concerned about her dependence on the practitioner. She may find herself unable to interpersonally communicate her struggles in the therapeutic relationship. The therapist, then, will need to be sensitive to nonverbal cues of communication. The client may be numbed or very anxious as a result of a paranoid fear that her therapist will victimize her by abandoning her. She may comply with the therapist and the demands of the therapeutic relationship. As she did as a child, she may attend to the adult's needs, care deeply for the therapist, and choose to protect him or her from her deepest rage and sorrow. She may even shield from the therapist the reality of her abuse experience and that her mother was actually the perpetrator. She may maneuver to comfort the therapist. She may lie to prevent the therapist from expressing negative feelings. She might believe that truth is expendable if it could get in the way of the relationship. This emotional entanglement of the client with her therapist provides a brilliant arena in which the client's story can unfold (Warme, 1996). The therapist is viewed not only as a substitute for life, the only one who listens and cares, but as a bridge to life. The feeling that someone truly hears, has immersed himself or herself in her inner world, is almost painful in its power to touch the mother-daughter-incest survivor whose story has historically been avoided, minimized, or exploited by many.

Given the compulsive, compliance characteristic of abused, traumatized persons, the client may cooperate with therapy by molding the self to the perceived needs of the therapist. The client may not wish to become confronted by what she is thinking and feeling, and therefore might engage in a humiliating appeal to achieve the comfort of knowledge that the therapist is not angry, disgusted, or about to terminate the therapy relationship (Crittendon, 1997). She may be expecting the same kind of obedience as she did from her parents who were constantly threatening to withdraw love or even abandon her if she criticized them or expressed noncompliance.

The adult survivor may protect her therapist from anger outbursts by denying their existence. She may turn the rage and hatred toward herself. These split-off rage responses may help the client maintain a positive image of the therapist and a tenuous attachment to him or her. She may act out her rage by engaging in self-destructive behaviors. Acting out can take the form of suicidal gestures and attempts, substance misuse, self-mutilation, sexual acting out, or anorexia or bulimia. This may be frustrating and frightening, producing a type of "helpless dread" in the therapist that can lead to defensively avoiding the client's problems or issues (Herman, 1992).

Trauma victims will present the clinician with more than the usual number of opportunities to sit through different transference-countertransference interactions. Mother-daughter incest survivors with multiple personality disorder represent the extreme in traumatic transference in that their identity may be highly fragmented with different components carried by different alters. Mother-daughter incest survivors, particularly those who have received a borderline personality diagnosis or who were abused as children, are likely to show heightened tendencies to terminate therapy early, to fail to attach to the therapist, or to act aggressively in therapy (Briere, 1989).

It is imperative that the clinician recognize that attachment is a dangerous process for any trauma victim. Certainly the mother-daughter incest survivor does not enter it blindly; entanglement is a dangerous as well as a life-giving function. Client hypervigilance is a problem and a fact of therapy with a mother-daughter incest survivor. She may become expert at reading the slightest nuance in the abuser, given that correct assessment of a perpetrator is so important to her personal safety (Briere, 1996). The therapist is watched constantly and is always on the brink of becoming an abusing or abused other (Davies and Frawley, 1994). The mother-daughter incest survivor feels an agonizing desire in the face of potential danger to find a witness to her trauma, and increasingly becomes dependent and reliant on the therapist as a caretaker. Therapists may find themselves inadequate to the task of meeting the survivor's yearning for protection, safety, and care.

The therapist may experience powerful, countertransferencial reactions to acting out client behaviors by feeling shocked, powerless, helpless, abused, and attacked. The therapist must address transferencial meanings embodied in the client's acting out. Not to do so evokes the image of the abuser who disclaimed the responsibility, or of the nonabusing parent who looked but did not see. Although it would be easy to deny the transference meaning of these acting out behaviors, it is important to address the client's vicious assaults on herself as well as the attacks on the therapist's goodness, caring, and effectiveness. At the same time, the therapist must acknowledge that much of the anger and rage projected toward him or her may be directed at the client's mother.

The therapist will need to guard against misreading the client's behavior as an attack, rather than understanding it as a defense. The therapist can encourage the survivor to give words to the depth of her anger and the profound terror associated with it. It is vital that the therapist recognize the terror, paralysis, hopelessness, and impotent rage that the client feels. Her anger is associated with power and a tremendous sense of loss of control. When the client finally expresses her anger, the therapist, while making every attempt not to minimize such anger, may be completely unprepared for the lack of reason and control (Pearlman and Saakvitne, 1995).

Once the survivor enters therapy, negative feelings about the clinician are often acted out. The client may report that her therapist disappointed her and made things worse. The client may feel betrayed by her therapist who encourages her to face situations rather than leave them untouched. She may feel betrayed by her therapist who encourages her to look at and work with memories of the abuse. She may feel pushed into participation, into revisiting the trauma of her abuse experience, and that the therapist did not warn her about the depth of feeling that would accompany reexposure. She may blame the clinician for stripping her of her defenses, leaving her emotionally vulnerable, aware, and alone. She may question the integrity of the clinician and ask why he or she would want to work with a mother-daughter incest survivor. She may accuse the therapist of being a seducer or seductress who gets off on abuse stories. She may attempt power and control in the therapeutic process in the form of invalidating the therapist. At this time, the therapist may question his or her own motives for working with survivors. He or she may feel abusive and unnecessarily voyeuristic.

The mother-daughter incest survivor needs to believe that her therapist also believes in the actuality of her trauma, and more important, in her experience of incest at the hands of her mother. The therapist must understand the problems of the mother-daughter incest survivor and give full credence to the childhood experiences she describes. He or she must understand that trauma attacked the coherence, reality testing, and worldview of the victim. He or she must empathetically recognize both the client's unequivocal yearning for love and protection and also the violent feelings toward her mother which may be directed toward the therapist. He or she must comprehend that people in helping roles frequently experience direct feelings from clients that are actually meant for parents or others in the client's life.

Female practitioners working with mother-daughter incest survivors need to be aware of transference issues, particularly in terms of anger toward the mother. The female counselor will need to be open to the exploration of anger, rage, and mistrust that is directed toward her. She will need to be receptive to the possibility of nonangry ambivalent feelings that the client may experience toward her mother. The male therapist may need to be open to feelings of anger and mistrust directed toward him because the client's father coperpetrated against her, or did not protect her, or perhaps was emotionally or physically absent in her life. Feelings, fears, defenses, and reactions, both positive and negative, may characterize other relationships that the client has with significant figures in her life.

The therapeutic relationship may be viewed by the client as causing anxiety, distrust, and criticism. The therapist's task will be to assist the client to grasp that much of her present resentment stems from the past mistreatment at the hands of her mother. The client needs to be reminded that it may be unproductive to continue fighting old battles. The client must come to realize that, with the therapist's support, the situation can be reversed, and that she has the power to change, to reject old beliefs and behaviors. She can now readily express overt gratitude, affection, and admiration and see the therapist in a more positive light. Anger, criticism, and dissatisfaction may dissipate to the point where the therapist is idealized.

In summary, the client may shift during the process of therapy from treating her therapist as though he or she was one of her parents to behaving toward the therapist in the way that one of her parents had treated her. The child who was subjected to hostile threats in childhood may use hostile threats to her therapist. Sexual advances from a parent may reappear as sexual advances to the therapist. The therapist needs to prepare for intensely hostile and sexualized transference and for emotional vicissitudes that are unpredictable and confusing for client and therapist alike. Both male and female practitioners will need to deal with transference issues and maintain professional boundaries within the therapeutic relationship. Learning to anticipate transferencial behaviors from the client may prove to be an important strategy in helping the therapist to be effective and to maintain a degree of control and even minimize the effects that transference reactions have on him or her. Therapists may react to the client's transferences, especially when working with the client's shame. In particular, those who are abuse survivors themselves, will need to understand they are subject to facing more of their own shame, a reminder that they are never completely finished as human beings (Fossum and Mason, 1986).

In the recovery process for the mother-daughter incest survivor, the therapist becomes the client's ally, placing all the resources of knowledge, skill, and experience at the client's disposal. The responsibility of the therapist is to use his or her position of power to foster the client's recovery, resisting all temptations to dominate or victimize the client. This promise is central to the integrity of the therapeutic relationship, and of particular importance to clients who have already suffered from exploitative exercises of power and control. Trauma clients, particularly those with a history of parental nonsupport and abuse, will not explore their feelings unless therapist attachment is trusted. The therapist, by keeping attachment issues at the forefront, is more likely to negotiate boundaries successfully while recognizing the enormous emptiness and terror that a perceived threat to attachment can bring to the mother-daughter incest survivor. Rigid boundaries interfere with client efforts to attach yet remain separate and to internalize the therapist's benevolence (Pearlman and Saakvitne, 1995). The therapist working with the mother-daughter incest survivor must realize that the client may have limited ability to "hold on" to a therapeutic relationship, or to any relationship for that matter. The therapist can err by taking over responsibility for the client's emotional safety, thereby obscuring the goals of therapy for client change and self-directed learning.

# Chapter 18

# Countertransference

Clinicians inevitably experience strong positive and negative feelings about their clients. Countertransference is defined by Dalenberg (2000) as "conflict-based emotional reactions to the client and all emotional reactions and related behaviors by the therapist" (p. 4). Countertransferential feelings involve all emotional reactions, conscious and unconscious, toward the client within the process of therapy as well as biased therapist behaviors that are based on life experiences and learning (Bouchard et al., 1995; Briere, 1989). Therapists are forced to face their own life cycle events, ghosts, and unfinished business from their family of origin. Therapists must examine their attitudes and beliefs about childhood sexual abuse before embarking on a therapeutic journey with a sexual abuse survivor.

The therapist feels and displays emotional reactions toward the traumatized client, the trauma material, and the transference dynamics displayed by the client. These feelings and actions on the part of the therapist in trauma treatment, a phenomenon called "traumatic countertransference" or "vicarious traumatization" (Pearlman and Saakvitne, 1995), have emotional significance to both the client and therapist and dramatically affect the course of therapy. Therapists are most likely to have strong negative and positive countertransference reactions to their traumatized clients than to other clients of similar ages and backgrounds. These feelings toward clients are confusing to many therapists. As a fellow human being, the helping professional may be outraged at a world that is hurtful and neglectful. The therapist may become emotionally overwhelmed as he or she experiences the same terror, rage, and despair as the client. Painful stories and human revelations are absorbed by the therapist. Hearing client stories of trauma may revive personal traumatic experiences, grotesque nightmares, and even symptoms of post-traumatic stress disorder within the therapist. Therapists may also have countertransferential reactions that are distinct from their feelings about the client. Therapist preexisting thoughts and beliefs about the trauma itself may affect the process of therapy profoundly. The practitioner may be personally repulsed or intimidated by the whole notion of a mother sexually abusing her daughter.

The therapist may identify with the mother-daughter incest survivor's rage. He or she may experience extremes of anger which may be directed at the perpetrator, at society in general, or at professional colleagues who lack understanding. The therapist may actually experience paranoid fear of the client's rage. He or she may experience profound grief, anguish, and despair and believe that he or she is in mourning along with the client. Repeated exposure to narratives of human capacity and cruelty profoundly challenges the therapist's basic faith and heightens his or her sense of personal vulnerability. It may leave him or her somewhat pessimistic, distrustful, and fearful of other people.

Working with any survivor is challenging for the therapist, but the issue of mother-daughter incest is likely to stretch the therapist beyond the parameters of his or her training, morals, and values. Working with mother-daughter incest survivors is likely to push the therapist to the limits of his or her mindfulness, creativity, and skills. The mother-daughter incest survivor has one of the most painful stories to tell. Countertransference is a regular and unavoidable occurrence for practitioners working with these survivors. The idea of a mother sexually abusing her daughter is likely to evoke in the therapist dreadful thoughts, feelings, images, and sensations. The therapist may experience emotional reactions toward the client which may have been evoked by some event in therapy or in the therapist's life. Both female and male therapists may easily transfer feelings that they have toward significant others in their lives to the mother-daughter incest survivor. They may be easily shocked, irritated, or repulsed by the issue of mother-daughter incest. They may be dealing with the client's fear that the therapist will vomit on the spot and throw her out of the office. They may feel intense anger toward the perpetrator. They may become depressed or overwhelmed after a session with their client, or highly emotional, perhaps lost in the client's world. They may drown in their own issues of abuse or neglect. The female practitioner may overidentify with the client, or overprotect her, thereby making it difficult to establish and maintain professional boundaries. Inevitably, the therapist will feel incompetent and hopeless, leading to an underestimation of his or her value, knowledge, and skill. He or she may lose faith in the power of the therapeutic alliance and may even lose sight of the client's strengths.

Practitioners working in the area of mother-daughter incest often describe their work as demanding, requiring energy, strength, availability, and vulnerability. Therapists who are themselves survivors may be particularly susceptible to countertransferential experiences. They may not remember their childhood abuse and begin to recall memories of their own trauma when they are working with survivors. For the therapist who is herself a mother-daughter incest survivor, countertransferential reactions may complicate her work and perhaps hinder the therapeutic alliance. For the female therapist, mother-daughter incest may be her most challenging issue to face. Issues concerning her own mother, such as abandonment or death, may leave the female therapist feeling vulnerable in her professional role.

Davies and Frawley (1994) use a relational approach integrated with a psychoanalytic perspective to describe four paradigms of transferential/countertransferential reactions between the client and the practitioner. This approach has real implications to the dual roles of survivor and practitioner and can be utilized to understand possible relational paradigms that may unfold between the mother-daughter incest survivor and her therapist. The therapist must be willing and able to work with these powerful and rapidly shifting paradigms commonly found in treatment of survivors:

1. the unseen, neglected child;
2. the sadistic abuser and the helpless enraged victim;
3. the idealized rescuer and the entitled child; and
4. the seducer and the seduced.

The mother-daughter incest survivor is often dependent and trusting of her therapist, an adult, with the horrible truth about the abuse she endured as a child. Within the therapeutic process, she risks reliving the trauma of the abuse. It is at this point in the process that the abused child ego state leads or directs the therapeutic triad (adult client, abused child self, and therapist) to the memory/affect bank of the trauma (Davies and Frawley, 1994). During this phase in the therapeutic process, the therapist, while encouraging the client to work through her tremendous pain and loss, is certainly challenged to withstand his or her client's despair and the limitations of his or her own ability to alleviate suffering.

The client may look to the therapist to make up for all the grief and suffering, to make sense of her experiences, and to integrate for her that which is fragmented. At the same time, the mother-daughter incest survivor fears the therapist's ability to make explicit the chaos and confusion as a result of her victimization at the hands of her mother. Part of her wishes to be left in peace. Part of her is enraged with the therapist, feeling victimized and abused by this ineffective intruder who sadistically enjoys stories of violent sexual abuse. The helpless, enraged victim may view the therapist as one more adult who will ultimately betray or abuse her, as being inexperienced, naïve, and ineffective. The therapist may countertransferentially experience corresponding feelings of being too intrusive, voyeuristic, abusive, ineffective, and needing to rescue the client.

The literature on the treatment of trauma addresses the likelihood that a client will accuse his or her therapist of "malfeasance, of covertly exploiting the client for his/her own narcissistic gratification" (Spiegel and Spiegel, 1978, p. 72). Mother-daughter incest survivors may frequently attack or accuse, thereby provoking defensive responses in the therapist. The phenomenon of repetition compulsion represents a pattern that is familiar and upsetting to any trauma therapist who is frightened and frustrated by the propensity for self-endangerment in the trauma client. The therapist faces emotionally challenging dilemmas: managing countertransferential hostility while retaining a hold on his or her own true self in the force of continued relational information that he or she is evil, dangerous, or a potential abuser. The therapist is constantly at risk of compassion fatigue and emotional exhaustion for caring for his or her client who is constantly at risk of physical or psychic destruction. To protect the self from this fatigue and psychic disequilibrium is one of the constant demands the therapist faces, often culminating in acting out countertransferentially (Stamm, 1995).

Provocative behavior, persistent boundary violation, self-endangerment, and suicidality on the part of the survivor is likely to press the therapist to the breaking point. At some point, the therapist may decide to confront the client. Sudden shifts by the therapist from tolerance to confrontation are reported in the literature to have positive effects. It is important to note, however, that extreme negative responses after a history of benevolence are likely to shock the client into silence and obedience (Carlson, 1997).

Therapy may be best described as a juggling act, a balancing act wherein the therapist delicately maneuvers between client dependability and moving too quickly, thereby overwhelming the client. The therapist will be challenged to address these manifestations or plethora of transferences while being open to the differences and disagreements between ego states. The therapeutic task is a difficult one because the adult client and abused child often work against each other with mutual hostility, mistrust, and resentment. A goal of therapy will be to have the adult nurturing, respecting, and parenting the neglected traumatized child. As the adult incorporates the traumatic memories, affects, and fantasies borne alone by the child, she recognizes the strength and resiliency of her child self. Hopefully, the abused child ego will learn to respect the ambition, decisiveness, thinking capabilities, and independence of her adult counterpart. In time, the mutual hatred and mistrust abate so that the adult and child grieve together the loss of fantasized good parents and an unmarred childhood. Concurrently, the adult client may rediscover the playfulness, creativity, and spontaneity long split off and held by the dissociated child self.

Ultimately, through the therapist's patience, consistent acceptance and interpretation of memories, feelings, fantasies, transferences, and countertransferences, the two ego states grow toward mutual understanding, respect, and affection. As these ego states integrate and the abused child cannot be found anymore, the therapist may countertransferentially grieve the departure of the child ego state. The therapist may grieve a loss of opportunity to be paternal, to protect, to rescue fantasies often elicited by the child's fragility and brokenness (Davies and Frawley, 1994). The therapist will need adequate support to bear this grief.

At times, the client may enact emotional coldness, rejection, and unavailability in the therapeutic process by becoming hostile to interpersonal engagement sought by the therapist. She may accuse the therapist of being demanding and of bothering her. She may appear bored, disdainful, and narcissistically preoccupied. As if identifying with her neglectful mother, she treats her own vulnerability, emotional needs, and affect states with the same cold neglect that she heaps on the therapist. She may view herself as weak and verbally berate herself much the same as her mother dismissed her feelings and yearnings to be cared for. Countertransferencially, the therapist may experience himself or herself as unseen, unwanted, unimportant, and disconnected with the client. He or she may feel frustrated, enraged, inadequate, and ultimately depressed in his or her struggle to connect with the client. He or she may give up, withdraw concern and interest in the client, and even appear unempathic. The therapist may blame the client for failure to adequately assess and respect his or her feelings. The therapist may frankly hate the client at times and hope that she withdraws from therapy.

A relational paradigm may exist, then, wherein both therapist and client experience themselves and each other as victim and victimizer. Both feel intruded upon, exposed, and penetrated. Both parties may protect themselves and avoid real engagements with each other. The client may feel entitled to extra attention, extra sessions, between session phone calls, and lengthened sessions. Clients often have strong reactions to changes or inconveniences that therapists may view as insufficient, such as a change in office location or a need to reschedule.

Client ambivalence about attachment can be extremely disconcerting and disheartening to the therapist who is unaccustomed to client experience of attachment as dangerous and yet necessary for survival. This ambivalence looks like an addiction and an allergy to closeness, and often leads to rapid vacillations in transference reactions. The therapist may find himself or herself in repeated boundary negotiations, feeling besieged by requests for intimacy one moment and accused of intrusion the next (Waites, 1993). Countertransferencially, the therapist, feeling caught between victim and perpetrator roles, may become challenged to identify as a caring individual. He or she may feel judgmental or skeptical about the client's story, minimize or rationalize the abuse, and feel contempt for the client's helplessness. She may feel disgust at the client's behavior, especially when she fails to follow through with expectations. The therapist may experience anger at being expected to serve as the all-giving parent.

Reenactment of the dynamics of victim and perpetrator in the therapy relationship can become extremely complicated. Sometimes the therapist may feel as if he or she is the client's victim and often complains of feeling threatened, manipulated, or exploited. He or she may feel anxiety and dread about upcoming sessions. The therapist may feel overwhelmed by the demands for more and more (more time, more energy, more phone calls, etc.), and blame himself or herself for initiating this pattern. Feeling used, helpless, and furious, the therapist may extricate himself or herself from relating to the client. The therapist may experience aspects of the client's victimized self, assume the blame for the abuse, feel violated and enraged but helpless to do anything else but accede to the client's demands.

The cycle of defensiveness, rage, denial, and self-punishment may come to the forefront for the client. She often feels furious, used, and helpless, and experiences the therapist as a powerful person. She may feel ashamed and enraged at herself for mistreating another, after having been so badly abused herself as a child. Ultimately, the therapist may feel manipulated and even controlled by the client and so may unconsciously enact an intrusive, controlling role with the client. He or she may refuse to acknowledge mistakes, similar to the perpetrator who will not take responsibility, and make shaming responses to perceived client attempts to manipulate, escalating the problem.

When the client is acting out or being self-abusive, the therapist, not wanting to appear uninvolved like the client's parent(s), may intrude to stop or limit the acting out. He or she may hospitalize the client or enforce behavioral contracts. Through acting out, the client may taunt or test the therapist to see if he or she will abandon the client. Yet throughout this phase, the client wants the therapist to gain control of her functioning. When the client acts out, the therapist may find himself or herself reacting with maternal/paternal feelings of caring, mild annoyance, or dismay at the client for her lack of coping skills, self-mastery, and self-worth. The therapist may also feel disturbed and disoriented by the client's projective identification and paralyzed and impotent as a therapist. He or she often feels beaten up by the client's relentlessness of self-mutilation and suicidal gestures. It is not uncommon for the therapist to feel afraid to confront these client behaviors for fear of escalation. To both the therapist and the client, these behaviors may feel like violence, intrusiveness, seduction, and betrayal.

Throughout therapy with any sexual abuse survivor, and perhaps more so with a mother-daughter incest survivor, the therapist may find himself or herself powerfully drawn into enacting the role of omnipotent, all-giving rescuer. He or she may want to save the broken child, the acting-out adolescent, or the adult survivor. This counter-transference may be especially potent when the client and/or thera-pist mourns the loss of childhood and of the fantasized good parents (Davies and Frawley, 1994). In the role of rescuer, the therapist may overly advocate for the client and assume too much personal respon-sibility for the client's life as a defense against the client's feelings of unbearable helplessness. In so doing, the therapist may imply that the client is not capable of deciding for herself of acting on her own be-half. The more the therapist accepts the idea that the client is helpless and dependent, the more he or she perpetrates the traumatic transfer-ence, the worse the child's symptoms become and the more she is disempowered. "Carried to the extreme, the therapist's defense against feelings of helplessness leads to a stance of grandiose specialness or omnipotence, and to an increased potential for corrupting the thera-peutic alliance" (Herman, 1992, p. 144).

Therapists may find themselves executing a delicate balancing act therapeutically. To the extent that they ignore or minimize the client's acting out or abusiveness, they recreate the unseeing, uninvolved par-ent. If they get locked countertransferencially in feeling victimized by the client, they may touch the client's shame or trigger feelings of guilt in the client. Both client and therapist wish to maintain a safe and benevolent world which leads them to struggle jointly with blame, shame, and responsibility in the relationship. Therapy can be a source of shame for the client because it encourages disclosure of unpleasant truths. The therapist may also feel shame for placing him-self or herself in the role of prosecutor or character assassin for some-one who came for comfort and compassion (Josephs, 1995). He or she can feel placed in the role of sadistic perpetrator as he or she par-ticipates in the recovery or processing of abuse memories. He or she may feel guilt and shame for triggering this painful period (Courtois, 1999).

Traumatized clients will feel unsafe in therapy about potential trig-gering of countertransference behaviors such as disapproval, disgust, dominance, and rejection brought on by client behaviors and history. Countertransference also presents the danger of confirming the cli-ent's trauma-related beliefs that the therapist is ashamed and dis-gusted by client behavior and that the therapist does not wish to be with the client. This undoubtedly contributes to feelings of profound despondence and hopelessness in the client. "The critical treatment element in this situation is for the therapist to hold onto the hope of a better life for the client, even when the client feels hopeless to do further work" (Dalenberg, 2000, p. 193).

Unique countertransference reactions can transform into shame when the therapist realizes that specific feelings toward the client are inappropriate. Sexual countertransference is experienced this way by a significant number of therapists. It is important for the therapist to understand that some types of child abuse, notably sexual abuse, lead the traumatized individual to fuse sexualization and affection, such that any positive relationship has strong sexual overtones. Other types of chronic childhood abuse can lead to a fusion of aggression and attachment, culminating in a connection to the therapist that feels both hostile and sexually toned. Therapists need to be encouraged to acknowledge this countertransference and tolerate their own shame without acting out punitively toward the client.

Understandably, sexualization by the client can be a trigger for sexual countertransference in the therapist. The therapist may experience voyeuristic excitement and intrigue, even sexual arousal which may force him or her to come to terms with his or her own capacity for evil (Herman, 1992). In a countertransference enactment, a therapist may feel empowered toward acts of sexual reparenting and attempting to salvage the sexual future of the client. Sexual encounters between client and therapist represent the most serious enactment of abusiveness/client victimization. The result, of course, is the tragic reabuse of the client. Any hope for future therapeutic work is destroyed, along with the integrity of the therapeutic boundaries.

Therapists may feel shame regarding unacceptable feelings from "bystander's guilt" for charging fees, especially when therapy is slow moving. They may feel shame about inadequacy in facing painful situations, at their unacceptable feelings and limitations, and at an enhanced awareness of a harsh, cruel world. It is vitally important for the therapist "to examine and highlight situational causes for shame, differentiating accusatory shame and the shame of the just, and containing angry responses to the client's humiliated fury. This will help minimize the harmful consequences of shame-related countertransference" (Dalenberg, 2000, p. 144).

In therapy, the client may identify with the perpetrator and seemingly smash progress and hope to bits. Such clients resist the most compelling enticements toward change. Identifying with the victim, the therapist experiences the despair and deflation once held by the victimized child. The therapist is further challenged by the extent to which the client's transference reactions are enacted rather than verbally identified and processed. It is the therapist's willingness to embrace and enact the relevant transferencial and countertransferencial positions that eventually allows the client to identify, tame, and integrate long split-off parts of her self and object worlds.

The therapist is responsible for acknowledging all aspects of countertransference in therapy with mother-daughter incest survivors. The therapist who is willing to own countertransference feelings is able to help the client learn to have faith in her own emotional perception. Countertransference disclosure models willingness to critically analyze internal experience. It is a necessary tool for demonstrating therapist credibility and genuineness, which is even more critical with clients whose traumas were delivered at the hands of attachment or authority figures (Dalenberg, 2000).

Chronic doubts in the reliability of their own perceptions appear to be the fate of many mother-daughter incest survivors and other chronic trauma victims. Countertransference withdrawal or avoidance on the part of the therapist can further undermine the client's sense of reality. For trauma clients whose past experience involved distortion and denial of physical and emotional reality, countertransference disclosure can help the client become more enlightened about her effect on other people and her contributions to intimate interactions. It can aid the mother-daughter incest survivor to move toward increased acceptance of others' emotions and to learn that low doses of negative affect from an attachment figure can be tolerated.

> Disclosure of anger or hostility can diminish client guilt and paranoia by making apparent the actual impact of her behavior. Disclosures can diminish the client's envy and establish the therapist's humanity because the client need not feel alone in her susceptibility to hostility. (Epstein, 1994, p. 175)

Creating a safe environment mandates attention to the actual countertransference of the therapist and to expected countertransference from the client's perspective. It mandates that the therapist guard against countertransference disclosures that are poorly disguised hostility, that distract self or client from painful material or attempt to reclaim the therapist's ravaged self-image (Hedges et al.,

1997). Although therapists attempt to control and moderate their hostility, their anger may be communicated through mistimed disclosure or subtle withdrawal. Therapists may countermanipulate through withdrawal, wherein their manipulative clients are punished by withholding normal connections in therapeutic sessions. Countertransference explosion from the therapist who is stretched to the limits of compassion is also a real danger in therapy. The goal of countertransference management and disclosure of anger is to model "anger in connection"—the ability to feel and disclose anger that is corrective, to have the experience of another human being who is willing to care despite his or her anger, and to negotiate a better relationship. If the therapist can model anger within connection, the client can learn that relationships which contain but which are not ruled by conflict or hostility are possible (Dalenberg, 2000; Crittendon, 1997; Davies and Frawley, 1994).

The practitioner must constantly evaluate his or her role in the therapeutic process and if he or she is effectively coping with providing therapy. Feeling "stuck" in therapy may be related to some unfinished business from the practitioner's family of origin. It may be related to feeling simultaneously angry and protective of the mother-daughter incest survivor because she may remind the practitioner of a younger sister, sibling, or even his or her own child. The therapist may suffer "witness guilt" for inducing or causing the client to reexperience trauma in the course of therapy and because he or she was spared the abuse. The female therapist may feel guilt for having a healthy relationship with her own mother. She may find it difficult to enjoy ordinary pleasures and comforts of life, and run the risk of ignoring her own legitimate interests, needs, and desires.

Trauma shatters the therapist's assumptions about this benevolent world. His or her emotional balance is constantly challenged when working with mother-daughter incest survivors. The therapist should expect to lose balance from time to time. The therapist, like the client, may defend against overwhelming feelings by withdrawal or by impulsive, intrusive action. The therapist may distance himself or herself professionally or frankly abandon the client. He or she may make rescue attempts, boundary violations, or attempts to control. He or she may doubt or deny the client's reality, dissociate or numb out, minimize or avoid the traumatic material. To the extent that the therapist feels endangered by the traumatic material, perhaps through parallels in his or her own past or present, it is more likely that the countertransference will be more extreme. This can lead to over-involvement and overemphasis on the trauma or to the unconscious avoidance of the material, mediated through disbelief and minimization (Davies and Frawley, 1994). The countertransference impulse to disbelieve may be strong, stemming from the therapist's protection against vicarious trauma, compassionate and empathic responses to client doubt, and incorporation of a societal disdain for victims. Belief and doubt will cycle in the therapist and client for complex sets of reasons related to the transference-countertransference matrix. The negotiation and acceptance of these cyclical changes is an important feature of therapy with mother-daughter incest survivors, as the participants work on emotionally challenging and stimulating material.

Working with mother-daughter incest survivors poses tremendous risk to the therapist's own psychological health. Therapists may experience symptoms of trauma associated with being victimized (Courtois, 1988; Briere, 1989) and may respond with a post-traumatic stress disorder-like syndrome. Dalenberg reports that 40 percent of therapists who work with traumatized clients display post-traumatic stress disorder symptoms. Suppressing their countertransference feelings can put them at risk for dissociative symptoms in which their suppressed feelings are acted out in therapeutic settings. They may experience high burnout and other negative symptoms such as shock, anger, anxiety, a sense of erosion of their self-esteem, feelings of hopelessness and helplessness, and feelings of incompetence. They may retaliate. They may feel increased irritability, free-floating anxiety, decreased ability to manage stress, increased difficulty in interpersonal relationships, depression, changes in social adjustment and in sexual functioning, as well as other psychological and physiological symptoms (Allen, 1996).

> Therapists often report uncanny, grotesque or bizarre imagery, dreams, or fantasies while working with survivors of severe early childhood abuse. They may have unaccustomed dissociative experiences including numbing and perceptual distortions, depersonalization and derealization, and at times may dissociate in concert with the client. (Herman, 1992, p. 146)

The therapist's adverse reactions, unless understood and contained, may seriously inhibit therapy and disrupt professional relationships. The therapist will require ongoing support systems to deal with these intense emotions. The practitioner must have colleagues available for support and advice since working with mother-daughter incest survivors in isolation may be particularly detrimental to all involved parties. The practitioner is encouraged to make use of consultation. A supportive environment of consultation will enable the practitioner to learn about himself or herself and to become more aware of his or her own missing pieces. The support system, which might include a supervisory relationship or a peer support group, should include a safe, structured, and regular forum for reviewing technical or intellectual concerns related to therapy with the client as well as emotional reactions. Therapists need to find a reliable, supportive network that understands their work so as to guard against their world narrowing where they feel they are the sole persons who really understand the clients. As they feel increasingly isolated and helpless, a professional support system reminds the therapist of his or her own realistic limitations and insists that self-care is just as important as the care given to others (Herman, 1992).

Support groups for the practitioner can prevent burnout and provide self-care. The following strategies may prove effective for the therapist working with mother-daughter incest survivors (Allen, 1996):

1. Be aware of personal and professional biases toward the issue of mother-daughter incest.
2. Strive to build and maintain competence.
3. Strive to anticipate and decrease burnout.
4. Obtain support and advice from other professionals/clinicians.
5. Be open to feedback from fellow practitioners.
6. Be realistic with goals and objectives with this particular population.
7. Avoid social isolation.
8. Measure successes in smaller increments.
9. Anticipate transferential behaviors from the client.

In summary, the therapist needs to be cognizant of countertransferential reactions related to his or her attitudes or experiences with trauma. Similar to the client, the therapist may be besieged by frightening countertransferential experiences and projective identification. This may challenge the therapist's willingness to hang in there with the client. He or she may feel the urge to disengage, withdraw, self-protect, or cancel therapeutic work. The therapist needs to recognize his or her own feelings of panic, ineffectiveness, and inadequacy and use the countertransference experience to refrain from emotionally abandoning the client. He or she will need to guard against compassion fatigue, which results in part from the strain of inhibiting strong and pressing emotion. This fatigue may be manifested as irritability or hostile interpretation. Through knowledge that projective identification will be an important component of the work, the therapist will be less likely to bolt or withdraw into self-protection which would ultimately hinder or threaten continued therapeutic success. He or she will need to understand that anger and hostility is a major problem in traumatized populations and a major counterreaction in trauma therapists. He or she must be cognizant of the fact that hostile interactions between therapist and client are predictive of poor long-term outcome.

Transference and countertransference reactions are inevitable. Their shifts are rapid and confusing. The therapist may feel completely bewildered by the rapid fluctuations in the client's moods or style of relating. The intensity of the transference often feels coercive to the therapist, and he or she may blame the client for this perceived coercion. The therapist may fear being misunderstood, wishing to appear compassionate and to avoid further pain. The client may worry about scrutiny of her past and present life for fear of discovery of a major character flaw or a set up for an accusation or confrontation. Hence both the client and the therapist share discomfort that they may rupture the therapeutic alliance. The intensity of transference and countertransference can overwhelm both participants and interfere with the development of a good working relationship. It is the therapist's ability to assume, enact, observe, and make explicit all the relational stances throughout the therapeutic dyad without being locked into any particular role or paradigm that moves treatment along.

The practitioner must give much attention to the issue of countertransference, in particular to steps that will assist and prepare him or her to deal with the issue. Countertransference may include avoidance, attraction, and attachment. Helplessness in the client may arouse parallel feelings of helplessness in the therapist. Certain protections are required for the safety of both client and therapist, and the two most important guarantees of safety are the goals, rules, and boundaries of the therapy contract and the support system of the therapist. Careful attention to the boundaries of the therapeutic relationship provides the best defense against extreme, unmanageable transference and countertransference reactions. Setting and maintaining clear boundaries is critical to successful therapy and to assist the therapist to guard against a pull to engage in a dual relationship with the client.

Finally, therapy with mother-daughter incest survivors requires great courage on the part of the client and an equal measure of honesty and courage on the part of the therapist.

> The volatility of the clients, the depth of yearning produced or awakened by the transference, the rigidity of repetitive patterns, and the frequency of the need for difficult boundary negotiations between client and therapist can all combine to exhaust the therapist, and contribute to a therapeutic impasse. (Dalenberg, 2000, p. 146)

Ways through this impasse include consultation, countertransference disclosure, careful attention to countertransference urges to blame or shame the client, and commitment to listen without defensiveness and with shared pain to the client's agony. It is critical that the therapist respect the bravery of the mother-daughter incest survivor as she breaks her silence and asks to be believed.

Chapter 19

# Theoretical Frameworks and Treatment Approaches

The therapist will need to draw from a number of theoretical frameworks that will guide therapeutic action. These frameworks will affect the therapist's perception and direct him or her to attend subjectively to certain phenomena which might otherwise be overlooked (Polansky, 1986). They provide a viable explanation in terms of why the mother-daughter incest survivor behaves the way she does.

Because child abuse and neglect cause disruptions in attachment which contribute to relational difficulties and establishment of intimate relationships, the therapist working with the mother-daughter incest survivor will need to address attachment-related issues of trust and dependency. Until these are resolved in some fashion, other developmental tasks may remain partially or fully unresolved. Various other developmental theories can also provide a deeper understanding of the issues that need attention and resolution. Erikson's (1970) theory of personality development jibes nicely with Kegan's (1982) attention to identity formation. Narrative therapy can help the mother-daughter incest survivor to see potential for new answers, for life that is not problem saturated, and for new self stories. A new script that is competency-based and full in terms of a sense of identity can leave space for the mother-daughter incest survivor to perform another narrative (Kamsler, 1990; Gil, 1996).

Although the clinical literature can help us to understand the incest survivor and give us a terminology, it is no substitute for the process of letting the survivor experience her feelings. A psychological understanding of incest is not enough. The mother-daughter incest survivor needs to confront the emotional realities and come to terms with them, feel the pain of what happened and grieve for herself before she can heal. She will need to appreciate that she is not the only person to go through maternal perpetrated abuse. She will need to appreciate that others have come through it and feel stronger and happier. She will need help to avoid being gobbled up by her feelings. She will need help to conquer feelings of profound despair and helplessness. She will need validation of thoughts and feelings that have been denied all her life. Cognitive-behavioral strategies can assist the mother-daughter incest survivor rectify thinking errors and affective deregulation, gain new perspectives on her problems, correct defective cognitions, and increase behavioral competencies.

The counseling relationship can serve as a powerful tool in helping the mother-daughter incest survivor find an alternate path toward fulfillment and toward beginning to change self-destructive thoughts and behaviors. Through therapy, the mother-daughter incest survivor can take inventory of the parts of her thoughts and feelings that were forced on her by abuse and dismiss them to make room for herself. The therapist can encourage the mother-daughter incest survivor to take possession of herself, to claim her experience, her thoughts, and her feelings for herself. She can be encouraged to love and hold the child within who was brutally wounded by her mother, to believe in her and defend her. She can be encouraged to hold the little girl tight while letting her cry, feel hurt, and express anger.

The therapist can draw on trauma theory because it fosters the notion that unresolved trauma can cause behavioral reenactments, compulsive behaviors, post-traumatic stress disorder (PTSD), and debilitating physiological responses. The trauma-specific phase of treatment, which is undertaken cautiously and purposely, focuses on the traumatic aspects of the abuse and brings them into conscience awareness with the goal of integrating the material in a less-fragmented manner. The mother-daughter incest survivor who has been traumatized by her abuse experience often has failed to examine and process the traumatic material and bring closure to her past abuse experience. In order for her to proceed, she will need to acknowledge the facts and repercussions of the abuse, release some of the feelings associated with the trauma that may have been unexpressed, examine a range of feelings toward her mother and other nonprotective family members or caretakers, and make cognitive reassessments of the abuse (why it happened, who was responsible, etc.). Beliefs that were generated during the trauma predicated on limited cognitions, dependency, intense fear, and feelings of disempowerment are frozen in time and must be addressed in a safe, structured environment. In therapy, only after a strong therapeutic relationship has developed and the client has a well-defined sense of self and a repertoire of coping strategies, can she address these beliefs, adequately gauge her pain thresholds, decrease her feelings of anxiety and pain, and generate a sense of internal and external supports. The therapist must feel assured that the client has personal power, i.e., she can agree or disagree to follow suggestions, and has the capacity to pace challenging material (Gil, 1996). By analyzing the traumatic past and bringing closure to it, the present and future feel more in the client's mastery.

Viewing the mother-daughter incest survivor through feminist, sociological, and multicultural perspectives is important as well. The reality from a feminist point of view is that women and children have longstanding histories of being devalued, disempowered, and victimized. Social norms allow or condone child abuse and neglect. For example, sexually exploited youth and the homeless are virtually ignored. Multiculturally, we must treat abused children within the context of their own culture, acknowledging that many cultures do not espouse formal therapy or the mental health system.

In counseling female victims (or offenders for that matter), the helper can begin by entering the world of these women, hearing their pain, anguish, and confusion and drawing on the women's own language and concepts to become the dominant mode of expression. An understanding of how sexism, racism, homophobia, and class oppression affects women is fundamental to effective work with them. Through listening and acknowledging the client's inner strength and resourcefulness, the therapist can help the client establish pathways toward fulfillment even after the most convoluted life stories are shared (van Wormer, 2001). The feminist practitioner can bring to the collaborative goal-setting process an intent to help women and other persons recover from the specific injuries of oppression, exploitation, and domination through their use of individual and collective power to reconstruct their realities.

## *POST-TRAUMATIC STRESS DISORDER*

Making use of the various theoretical frameworks just described can enable the practitioner to develop a strong therapeutic relationship that over time can provide a safe, rewarding, corrective, and reparative experience for the mother-daughter incest survivor. Always at the forefront of therapy is a mother-daughter incest survivor's sense of self as she learns to self-monitor, self-regulate, and develop behaviors that elicit more positive responses.

Mother-daughter incest survivors lose the capacity for effective regulation of emotional states due to post-traumatic stress disorder. As with other individuals who have been diagnosed with PTSD, specific emotions, images, sensations, and muscular reactions may have been imprinted on their minds. These traumatic imprints may be reexperienced months, years, even decades after the trauma transpired (Van der Kolk, 2002). Sufferers of PTSD behave as if they were living in the past because of their failure to transform and integrate sensory imprints associated with the trauma and their inability to realize that the feelings and actions are irrelevant to the present. The mind loses its flexibility to attach incoming sensory information to a whole range of associations. Instead, trauma becomes a gaping hole that connects all sensations. The process of dissociation, a characteristic of PTSD, which served as a defense at the time of the trauma, now occurs involuntarily in stressful situations, preventing them from integrating traumatic memories, putting the trauma behind them, and minimizing its impact. Fragmented sensory or emotional elements are triggered uninvited and do not fade with time. The entire neural net in which memory is stored is activated. Sensorimotor processes from the original trauma have not been assimilated and are easily triggered again and again. Certain sensations and emotions may surface as episodes of confusion, disorientation, freezing of thought processes, or total amnesia. Anniversary dates, people, places, objects, and emotional situations that remind the sufferer of the original trauma can serve as triggers. At the mercy of their sensations, physical reactions, and emotions, it is difficult for PTSD sufferers to modulate how they feel; they lose the capacity for effective regulation of emotional states. When confronted with elements of the original trauma(s), they have psychophysiological reactions and neuroendocrine responses that reflect their having been conditioned to respond to certain traumatic reminders. Their biological systems are activated as if they were traumatized all over again. The fundamental dynamic underlying PTSD is a cycle of reexperiencing the trauma, followed by attempts to bury memories and feelings associated with the trauma. Exploration of the nature of the abuse is usually accompanied by very intense emotions as repressed memories are released. Repetitive intrusions of a cognitive nature may occur such as nightmares, hallucinations, recurrent images, or obsessive thoughts. They may experience uncontrollable weeping, fear, or panic. Sufferers could exhibit behavioral aspects such as compulsive talking about the trauma, bodily reenactments, or artistic renderings. Lacking the capacity to soothe themselves, PTSD sufferers rely on impulsive actions to regulate their internal homeostasis, such as fight-or-flight, or pathological self-soothing, such as self-mutilation, bingeing, starving, drug or alcohol use, running away, reckless spending, promiscuity, reckless driving, and even child abuse (Bronson, 1989; Van der Kolk, 2002; Shapiro, 1995).

Because PTSD consists of a frozen sensory world, the therapeutic challenge is to open the client's mind to new possibilities so that she can encounter new experiences with openness and flexibility rather than interpreting the present as a continuous reliving of the past. The brain must be deconditioned from interpreting innocuous reminders as a return of the trauma. One central challenge when treating PTSD is how to help sufferers process and integrate traumatic material without making them feel traumatized once more.

Eye movement desensitization and reprocessing (EMDR) is a revolutionary method of psychotherapy that is well researched and validated as a way to treat PTSD and certain types of mental conditions and disorders. EMDR improves real-life performance in a wide range of challenging situations and causes the brain to learn much more quickly than usual, making possible the rapid recovery from the effects of acute or chronic psychological trauma. EMDR works with a wide variety of problems not previously thought to be trauma related such as substance abuse, depression, bipolar disorder, schizophrenia, anxiety disorders, acting-out problems in children and adolescents, sleep disorders, anger management, chronic pain, and somatization disorders (Shapiro, 2002).

EMDR enables the client to access old toxic memories of early trauma and rapidly and effectively reprocess and integrate them via bilateral stimulation. The client is asked to focus intensely on the emotions, sensations, and meaning associated with her traumatic experience while participating in rhythmic bilateral stimulation of one of the senses via flashing lights, waving fingers, hand taps, or alternating tones. The theory is that the stimulation of both right and left hemispheres somehow unblocks traumatic memories that have been frozen at a time when the client was unable to process the over-whelming emotions associated with the traumatic event (Pinker, 2002). Linking traumatic memories with adaptive, realistic interpre-tations and a more distanced emotional outlook seems to be EMDR's desired end point. The client is asked to find an imaginary safe place to retreat to if therapy becomes too upsetting. She is asked to conjure up a painful "target experience" while rating her level of emotional discomfort. Reprocessing comes when the client focuses on several sets of bilateral stimulation, whether this is watching the therapist re-peatedly wave his/her fingers from left to right, looking at flashing lights, listening to alternating tones, or feeling the therapist's alternat-ing hand taps on the client's palms or knees. The sets of bilateral stimulation incite associations, feelings, and memories that sponta-neously float to the surface. The client is encouraged to rate her dis-comfort during the process of uncovering memory, gradually associ-ating more adaptive interpretations of past events. Guided imagery and cognitive-behavioral interventions can enable the client to gain ac-cess and insight into what had previously been locked within. Free associative processes are released, giving the client very rapid access to material that she had not consciously considered as being relevant to her present quandaries. This allows her to associate current painful life experiences to prior life events that have been successfully mas-tered (Pinker, 2002). The client is much more articulate about the im-ages and thoughts that come to her awareness during EMDR.

The practice of EMDR seems to accomplish therapeutic action while clients remain in a relative state of speechlessness. Intense physiological reactions and psychological distress may disappear following a few sessions of EMDR. An event, which initially seemed to be re-lived with timeless energy, may become relegated to the past. The client is able to transform her experiences, integrate her memo-ries of what happened to her, and move on with her life. She can form new associations that do not lead to reliving the past. She can physi-cally experience new possibilities by welcoming and allowing split-off bodily feelings to run their course.

Trauma is not primarily imprinted on people's consciousness, but instead becomes deeply imbedded in their sensate experiences. Talk-ing and insight may help people regain a sense of mastery, but people's sensate experiences form the engines that drive traumatic reliving. The efficacy of EMDR as a therapy is relevant for the exploration of the basic underlying mechanisms of post-traumatic stress such as how trauma affects subcortical processes of emotion regulation, arousal modulation threat information, and memory processes. It sheds light on the fundamental question of how the mind integrates experience in such a way that it is prepared for future threat while being able to make a distinction between what belongs to the present and what belongs in the past.

## *AN INTEGRATED TREATMENT MODEL*

Assisting people to rapidly and effectively process traumatic sensations and emotions through bilateral eye movements is a remarkable step toward exploring new avenues of helping people move beyond the tyranny of their traumatic histories. Working with an experienced EMDR therapist can help the client move through dissociation, more clearly recall events, resolve any painful feelings about her traumatic past and any other abusive events in her personal history. Obstacles are removed for the client and control is returned to her body and mind. Seldom used alone as a tool, EMDR is a way of allowing a brain disorder to correct itself and to solve problems in a context of various methods of practicing psychotherapy.

The therapist must be open to the formulation of a comprehensive treatment plan, based on the clinical presentation of the client, which addresses behavioral and emotional problems. The therapist will need to consider the relevance of an approach that addresses post-traumatic stress, a core effect of trauma (especially child sexual abuse), when working with mother-daughter incest survivors. The treatment of PTSD is complicated due to the wide range of symptoms and intricate psychobiologic features. He or she will need to embellish different treatment modalities (individual, family, group, psychopharmacologic therapy), which may be required at different points in the therapeutic process. He or she will need to be open to the potential for three branches of treatment that involve client education, pharmacotherapy, and psychotherapy.

Along with psychotherapy, pharmacotherapy has been shown to alleviate the three clusters of PTSD symptoms (reexperiencing, avoidance, and hypervigilance) as well as coexisting conditions such as depression and anxiety (Friedman, 1998; Matsakis, 1992). Selective serotonin reuptake inhibitors (SSRIs) may help reduce PTSD symptoms such as nightmares, recurring thoughts, and flashbacks, as well as hyperalert symptoms, the startle response, and sweating. Concurrent ADHD, and persistent insomnia accompanied by significant hyperarousal and reexperiencing symptoms may be treated with clonidine (Brady et al., 1995). Medication has not been found to help the PTSD sufferer cope with the avoidance of triggers. Medication must be accompanied with therapy in order for healing to occur.

In psychotherapy, attention is paramount to a wide range of issues including the effects on the family, education about the causes and symptoms of PTSD, recognition of cues or situations that trigger symptoms, treatment options, and clinical courses. The more the client learns about PTSD the more in control of her life she will feel. "Knowledge is the best antidote to fear" (Matsakis, 1992, p. 27). Relaxation techniques such as deep breathing or muscle relaxation can improve the client's coping mechanisms, extinguish the fear response, and foster relationships with others. Relaxation training may help the client learn to control fear and anxiety by systematically relaxing major muscle groups. Techniques to assist the client to remember as much of the trauma as possible and reconstruct it mentally (what Matsakis terms the "cognitive stage" of the healing process) include written exercises, exercises using prompts, e.g., pictures, storytelling, dancing, drawing, art therapy, talking to others, and reading. Cognitive-behavioral therapy can assist the client to examine and correct cognitive distortions and help her to gain control over intrusive reexperiencing symptoms. Positive self-talk can assist the client through a trigger situation. Hypnotherapy and stress inoculation training (systematic desensitization) are helpful against reexperiencing and avoidance symptoms. Anxiety management, massage, and play therapy may also be useful as treatment strategies. Assertiveness training and anger management can enable her to express her wishes, opinions, and emotions without alienating others. Group therapy can help the client experiment with, elaborate, integrate, and reinforce skills for fear reduction, affect regulation, avoidance, hyperarousal symptoms, and interpersonal engagement.

Finally, the therapist working with mother-daughter incest survivors will need to have the aptitude to guide a search for meaning, to recognize existential despair, to confront self-pity, and to reinforce recognition of one's responsibility for one's own life (Wilson and Raphael, 1993). He or she will need to see beyond any singular treatment modality. No matter what therapeutic approach is utilized, it is vital that the therapist recognize that each individual has a unique pathway to recovery. He or she must ensure that the client has the opportunity to make an informed choice among effective options. The client will need support during the "emotional stage of the healing process" (Matsakis, 1992) as she faces her memories, feels her emotions, and tries to work through them. Telling the details of the trauma and revisiting the terror can remove the grip of horror. She will need to feel the therapist's presence, the bond of mutual respect, the partnership in survival. Revisiting the trauma is painful, but it is necessary and unavoidable. As normalization restores a sense of dignity, as empowerment restores a will to endure, and as individuality restores a sense of mastery, clients do take responsibility to find the right answers for themselves.

# Chapter 20

# Conclusion

To understand incest and to help victims in their recovery process, helping professionals must acknowledge that women as well as men may sexually abuse their children. Therapists need to be open to the possibility of mother-daughter incest. Recent research clearly indicates that the experience of mother-daughter incest is traumatic for its victims. Due to their premature sexualization as children, the profound betrayal of trust because their perpetrator was their mother, and the taboo and enforced silence which has historically surrounded the phenomenon of mother-daughter incest, the women inevitably experience deep wounding that leaves a devastating impact on their lives. The trauma of the abuse experience robs the mother-daughter incest survivor of a sense of power and control. She feels unsafe in her body. Her emotions and cognitions feel out of control. She often feels unsafe in relation to other people. Her abuse experience at the hands of her mother severely threatens both mind and body.

Since betrayal of trust is a major cause of wounding for the mother-daughter incest victim, the therapist must pay particular attention to the therapeutic alliance and to the establishment and maintenance of healthy boundaries between client and therapist so that the client does not face further violation. A lengthy period of time may be required to establish the therapeutic alliance. Because of the severity of the abuse, its devastating impact on the developmental process, and the time required to establish a therapeutic relationship, therapy may be long-term. Because the incest wound is particularly deep, mother-daughter incest survivors may respond slowly to treatment.

Many mother-daughter incest survivors will turn to therapy with clear goals of achieving a healthier life, and overcoming their profound feelings of disconnection, isolation, and alienation. It is vitally important that the process of therapy not repeat exploitation and betrayal of the survivor. Therapy must address her safety concerns in her life domains and provide a secure environment where the mother-daughter incest survivor can disclose and feel believed, protected, accepted, and valued throughout her terrifying descriptions of pain and shame. The therapist needs to hear what the survivor needs to say, believe it, and provide human contact, warmth, and engaged conversation in therapy.

The guiding principle of recovery for the mother-daughter incest survivor, not unlike other trauma victims, is to restore power and control to the victim. The mother-daughter-incest survivor must be allowed to carefully uncover at her own pace her secrets that have been buried for years. They are complex and tenacious and must be approached cautiously and thoughtfully. The therapist's responsibility is to discover ways to create a relatively safe environment in which the client can disclose the details of her traumatic past within a genuine relationship. Within this one-to-one relationship with a therapist, the heart of darkness can open (Bepko and Krestan, 1990).

For me, the most compelling aspects of their stories are the coping strategies and processes of recovery these women used. Many of these women resorted to some form of creativity to work through their pain. By engaging in the creative process, they faced their anguish by incorporating pain with the jubilation of bringing something new to life. Through art, revisiting and confronting their trauma helped them gain strength, restore their self-esteem, and find meaning in their life. Despite the pain of their experience, they struggled, persevered, and resisted defeat. They needed to regroup and make sense of what happened to them. They were challenged to integrate their experience into the life they still have, but a life that had been changed forever. They discovered meaning and purpose by tapping into their inner strength, redirecting their thinking and priorities, opening up new roads, new skills, new visions of the world and their place in it.

Breaking the silence marks the beginning to the end of secrets and isolation. Building a new life for the mother-daughter incest survivor will be a slow process requiring a lifetime of dedication and consistent work. Through connecting with others, whether in one-to-one therapy or group support, the mother-daughter incest survivor can feel believed and validated. Each encounter with people who are supportive will build her confidence and trust. Through sharing their stories, the social bonds that were destroyed by incest are mended, and the traumatic experience is given new meaning in the retelling. It becomes a gift to others.

The destruction of attachments as a result of her abuse experience must be addressed by interpersonal strategies that include the gradual development of a trusting relationship in therapy. Social alienation must be addressed through social strategies such as mobilizing the survivor's natural support systems, and introducing her to self-help organizations. Her important relationships will be reestablished, a coherent system of meaning and belief will be constructed that encompasses the story of her trauma and deepens and expands her integration of the meaning of her experience.

Because of the profound taboo against mother-daughter incest and the fact that research in the area is sparse, the topic of mother-daughter incest needs to be further explored. As a society, we can no longer deny the existence of mother-daughter incest. Turning away from the fact that mothers can and sometimes do sexually abuse their daughters only betrays survivors further, keeps them shrouded in silence and shame, and trapped in fear and self-loathing. It hinders their ability to feel safe in the world, to heal, to feel in control of their lives, to survive. It contributes to their feelings of hopelessness and helplessness, that they are trapped with no place to go. It exacerbates their belief that they are only strays, unwanted orphans, who will remain for the rest of their lives unattached, unprotected, and unvalued. For human beings already suffering from mental and physical health issues, it makes suicide an attractive option.

The therapeutic alliance can make many things possible for the client. By listening with knowledge, skill, and empathy the therapist can provide the context of a positive relationship that sets the stage for healing disclosures, healthy boundaries, and mutuality of caring between the client and therapist. "In the course of successful therapy, it should be possible to recognize a gradual shift from unpredictable danger to reliable safety, from dissociated trauma to acknowledged memory, and from stigmatized isolation to restored social connection" (Herman, 1992, p. 155). The survivor will turn her attention from the tasks of recovery to the tasks of ordinary life. The best indices of trauma resolution are the survivor's capacity to take pleasure in her life and to engage fully in relationships with others.

# Bibliography

Abney, V. (1992). Transference and countertransference issues unique to long-term group psychotherapy of adult women molested as children. *Journal of Interpersonal Violence,* 7(4), 559-569.

Allen, J.G. (1996). *Borderline personality disorder: Tailoring the psychotherapy to the patient.* American Psychiatric Publishing.

Banning, A. (1989). Mother-son incest: Confronting a prejudice. *Child Abuse and Neglect,* 13, 563-570.

Baures, M. (1994). *Undaunted spirits: Portraits of recovery from trauma.* Philadelphia: The Charles Press, Publishers.

Bennett, M. (1993). *The child as psychologist: An introduction to the development of social cognition.* New York: Harvester Wheatsheaf.

Bepko, C. and Krestan, J. (1990). *Too good for her own good.* New York: Harper & Row.

Bilker, L. (1993). Male or female therapists for eating-disordered adolescents: Guidelines suggested by research and practice. *Adolescence,* 28(110), 393-422.

Blanchard, G. (1987). Male victims of child sexual abuse: A portent of things to come. *Journal of Independent Social Work,* 1(1), 19-27.

Bouchard, M., Normandin, L., and Seguin, M. (1995). Countertransference as instrument and obstacle: A comprehensive and descriptive framework. *Psychoanalytic Quarterly,* 44, 717-745.

Bowlby, J. (1982). *Attachment and loss,* Second edition. Volume 1: *Attachment.* London: The Hogarth Press.

Bowlby, J. (1988). *A secure base.* New York: Basic Books.

Boyd, C. (1989). Mothers and daughters: A discussion of theory and research. *Journal of Marriage and the Family,* 51, 291-301.

Brady, K.T., Soune, S.C., and Roberts, J.M. (1995). Sertraline treatment of comorbid posttraumatic-like stress disorder and alcohol dependence. *Journal of Clinical Psychiatry,* 56, 502-505.

Brassell, W. (1994). *Belonging: A guide to overcoming loneliness.* Oakland, CA: New Harbinger Publications, Inc.

Breckenridge, J. and Baldry, E. (1997). Workers dealing with mother blame in child sexual assault cases. *Journal of Child Sexual Abuse,* 6(1), 65-80.

Briere, J. (1984). *The effects of childhood sexual abuse on later psychological functioning.* Washington, DC: National Medical Center.

Briere, J. (1989). *Therapy for adults molested as children: Beyond survival.* New York: Springer.

Briere, J. (1996). *Therapy for adults molested as children: Beyond survival.* Second edition. New York: Springer.

Briere, J. and Runtz, M. (1986). Suicidal thoughts and behaviours in former sexual abuse victims. *Canadian Journal of Behavioural Science,* 18, 413-423.

Bronson, C. (1989). *Growing through the pain.* New York: Prentice-Hall.

Browne, A. and Finkelhor, D. (1986). Impact of child sexual abuse. *Psychological Bulletin,* 99, 66-77.

Browning, D. and Boatman, B. (1977). Incest: Children at risk. *American Journal of Psychiatry,* 134, 69-72.

Bureau of Justice Statistics (1997). Sex offenses and offenders: An analysis of data on rape and sexual assault. Washington, DC: U.S. Department of Justice.

Bureau of Justice Statistics (1999a). Juvenile arrests. Washington, DC: U.S. Department of Justice.

Bureau of Justice Statistics (1999b). Women offenders. Washington, DC: U.S. Department of Justice.

Carlson, E. (1997). *Trauma assessments: A clinician's guide.* New York: Guilford Press.

Chesney-Lind, M. (1997). *The female offender: Girls, women, and crime.* Thousand Oaks, CA: Sage Publications.

Chodorow, N. (1974). Family structure and feminine personality. In M.A. Rosaldo and L. Lamphere (Eds.), *Women, culture, and society* (pp. 43-66). Stanford, CA: Stanford University Press.

Chodorow, N. (1978). *The reproduction of mothering: Psychoanalysis and the sociology of gender.* Berkeley: University of California Press.

Courtois, C.A. (1988). *Healing the incest wound.* New York: W. W. Norton and Company.

Courtois, C.A. (1999). *Recollections of sexual abuse: Treatment principles and guidelines.* New York: W. W. Norton and Company.

Crittendon, P. (1997). Patterns of attachment and sexual behavior: Risk of dysfunction vs. opportunity for creative integration. In L. Atkinson and K. Zuckerman (Eds.), *Attachment and Psychopathology* (pp. 47-93). New York: Guilford Press.

Cuffe, S.E. and Frick-Helms, S.B. (1995). Treatment interventions for child sexual abuse. In G.A. Rekers (Ed.), *Handbook of child and adolescent sexual problems* (pp. 232-251). New York: Lexington Books.

Dalenberg, C. (2000). *Countertransference and the treatment of trauma.* Washington, DC: American Psychological Association.

Davies, J.M. and Frawley, M.G. (1994). *Treating the adult survivor of child sexual abuse.* New York: Basic Books.

Epstein, R. (1994). *Keeping boundaries: Maintaining safety and integrity in the psychotherapeutic process.* Washington, DC: American Psychiatric Press.

Erikson, E.H. (1970). *Childhood and society.* Harmondsworth, England: Penguin Books.

Evert, K. and Bijkerk, I. (1987). *When you're ready: A woman's healing from childhood physical and sexual abuse by her mother.* Walnut Creek, CA: Launch Press.

Finkelhor, D. (1979). *Sexually victimized children.* New York: The Free Press.

Finkelhor, D. and Browne, A. (1985). The traumatic impact of child sexual abuse: A conceptualization. *American Journal of Orthopsychiatry,* 55(4), 530-541.

Finkelhor, D., Hotaling, G., Lewis, I.A., and Smith, C. (1989). Sexual abuse and its relationship to later sexual satisfaction, marital status, religion, and attitudes. *Journal of Interpersonal Violence,* 4(4), 379-399.

Finkelhor, D. and Russell, D. (1984). Women as perpetrators. In D. Finkelhor and associates (Eds.), *Child sexual abuse: New theory and research* (pp. 171-185). New York: The Free Press.

Fischer, L. (1986). *Linked lives: Adult daughters and their mothers.* New York: Harper & Row.

Flax, J. (1978). The conflict between nurturance and autonomy in mother-daughter relationships and within feminism. *Feminist studies,* 4(2), 171-189.

Flax, J. (1989). *Thinking fragments: Psychoanalysis, feminism, and postmodernism in the contemporary west.* Berkeley: University of California Press.

Forward, S. and Buck, C. (1988). *Betrayal of innocence.* London: Penguin Books.

Fossom, M.A. and Mason, M.J. (1986). *Facing shame: Families in recovery.* New York: W. W. Norton and Company.

Friday, N. (1977). *My mother myself.* New York: Delacorte Press.

Friedman, M.J. (1998). Current and future drug treatment for posttraumatic stress disorder patients. *Psychiatry,* 28, 461-468.

Gelinas, D.J. (1983). The persisting negative effects of incest. *Psychiatry,* 46, 313-332.

Gil, E. (1995). *Systemic treatment of families who abuse.* San Francisco: Jossey-Bass.

Gil, E. (1996). *Treating abused adolescents.* New York: Guilford Press.

Gilbert, L. and Webster, P. (1982). *Bound by love: The sweet trap of daughterhood.* Boston: Beacon Press.

Gilligan, C. (1982). *In a different voice.* Cambridge, MA: Harvard University Press.

Goodwin, J. and Divasto, P. (1979). Mother-daughter incest. *Child Abuse and Neglect,* 3, 953-957.

Groth, A.N. (1982). The incest offender. In S.M. Sgroi (Ed.), *Handbook of clinical intervention in child sexual abuse* (pp. 215-239). Lexington, MA: D.C. Heath.

Hedges, L., Hilton, R., Hilton, V., and Candill, O. (1997). *Therapists at risk: Perils of the intimacy of the therapeutic relationship.* Northvale, NJ: Jason Aronson.

Herman, J. (1981). *Father-daughter incest.* Cambridge, MA: Harvard University Press.

Herman, J. (1992). *Trauma and recovery.* New York: Basic Books.

Hoagwood, K. (1990). Blame and adjustment among women sexually abused as children. *Women and Therapy,* 9, 89-110.

Hyde, N. (1986). Covert incest in women's lives: Dynamics and directions for healing. *Canadian Journal of Community Mental Health,* 5(2), 73-83.

Jacobs, M. (1998). Requiring battered women die: Murder, liability for mothers under failure to protect statutes. *Journal of Criminal Law and Criminology,* 88(2), 579-660.

Janoff-Bulman, R. (1979). Characterological versus behavioral self-blame: Inquiries into depression and rape. *Journal of Personality and Social Psychology,* 37, 1798-1809.

Janoff-Bulman, R. (1992). *Shattered assumptions.* New York: The Free Press.

Johnson, R.L. and Shrier, D. (1987). Past sexual victimization by females of male patients in an adolescent medical clinic population. *American Journal of Psychiatry,* 144(5), 650-652.

Jordan, J. V. and Surrey, J.L. (1986). *The self-in-relation: Empathy and the mother-daughter relationship.* Work in Progress. Wellesley, MA: Stone Center Working Paper Series.

Josephs, L. (1995). *Balancing empathy and interpretation: Relational character analysis.* Northvale, NJ: Jason Aronson.

Joyce, P.A. (1997). Mothers of sexually abused children and the concept of collusion: A literature review. *Journal of Child Sexual Abuse,* 6(2), 75-92.

Kamsler, A. (1990). Her story in the making: Therapy with women who are sexually abused in childhood. In M. Durrant and C. White (Eds.), *Ideas for therapy with sexual abuse* (pp. 9-36). Adelaide, Australia: Durwich Centre.

Kaplan, A.G. (1991). The "self-in-relation." *Women's Growth in Connection.* Work in Progress. Wellesley, MA: Stone Center Working Paper Series.

Kaplan, A.G., Gleason, N., and Klein, R. (1991). Women's self-development in late adolescence. *Women's Growth in Connection.* Work in Progress. Wellesley, MA: Stone Center Working Paper Series.

Karen, R. (1994). *Becoming attached: Unfolding the mystery of the infant-mother bond and its impact on later life.* New York: Warner.

Kegan, R. (1982). *The evolving self.* Cambridge, MA: Harvard University Press.

Knight, C. (1997). Critical roles and responsibilities of the leader in a therapy group for adult survivors of child sexual abuse. *Journal of Child Sexual Abuse,* 6(1), 21-37.

Kunzman, K.A. (1990). *Freedom from the tyranny of the past.* New York: Harper & Row.

Lanese, J. (1998). *Mothers are like miracles.* New York: Simon and Schuster.

LaSorsa, V. and Fodor, I. (1990). Adolescent daughters/midlife mother dyad. *Psychology of Women Quarterly,* 14, 593-606.

Littrell, J. (1998). Is the experience of painful emotion therapeutic? *Clinical Psychology Review,* 18, 71-102.

Lloyd, C. (1987). Working with the female offender: A case study. *British Journal of Occupational Therapy,* 50(2), 44-46.

Magrab, P. (1979). *Psychological management of pediatric problems.* Baltimore: University Press.

Maison, S.R. and Larson, N.R. (1995). Psychosexual treatment program for women sex offenders in a prison setting. *Nordisk Sexologi,* 13, 149-162.

Matsakis, A. (1992). *I can't get over it: A handbook for trauma survivors.* Oakland, CA: New Harbinger Publications, Inc.

Matthews, J., Mathews, R., and Speltz, K. (1991). Female sexual offenders: A typology. In M. Q. Patton (Ed.), *Family sexual abuse* (pp. 199-219). Newbury Park, CA: Sage Publications.

Mayer, A. (1983). *Incest: A treatment manual for therapy with victims, spouses, and offenders.* Holmes Beach, FL: Learning Publications.

McCarthy, L.M. (1986). Mother-child incest: Characteristics of the offender. *Child Welfare,* 65, 447-458.

Meiselman, K.C. (1978). *Incest: A psychological study of cause and effects with treatment recommendations.* San Francisco: Jossey-Bass.

Miller, A. (1976). *Toward a new psychology of women.* Boston: Beacon Press.

Miller, D. (1994). *Women who hurt themselves.* New York: Basic Books.

Miltenburg, R. and Singer, E. (1997). A theory and support method for adult sexual abuse survivors living in an abusive world. *Journal of Child Sexual Abuse,* 6(1), 39-63.

Office of Juvenile Justice and Delinquency Protection (1998). *Juvenile female offenders: A status of the states report.* October. Washington, DC: Office of Juvenile Justice and Delinquency.

Ogilvie, B. (1996). *Why didn't she love me?* Vancouver, British Columbia, Canada: Hazeldine Press.

Ogilvie, B. and Daniluk, J. (1995). Common themes in the experiences of mother-daughter incest survivors: Implications for counseling. *Journal of Counseling and Development,* 73, 598-602.

O'Hagan, K. (1989). *Working with child sexual abuse: A post-Cleveland guide to effective principles and practice.* Milton-Keynes, UK: Open University Press.

Pearlman, L. and Saakvitne, K. (1995). *Trauma and the therapist: Countersference and vicarious traumatization in psychotherapy with incest survivors.* New York: W. W. Norton and Company.

Pelletier, G. and Handy, L. (1986). Family dysfunction and the psychological impact of child sexual abuse. *Canadian Journal of Psychiatry,* 31, 407-411.

Pinker, S. (2002). The eyes may have it. *The Globe and Mail* (p. R6), June 25, 2002.

Polansky, N. (1986). There is nothing so practical as a good theory. *Child Welfare,* 65(1), 3-15.

Rhodes, G. and Rhodes, R. (1996). *Trying to get some dignity.* New York: Morrow and Company, Inc.

Rosencrans, B. (1997). *The last secret: Daughters sexually abused by mothers.* Brandon, VT: Safer Society Press.

Rubin, L. (1983). *Intimate strangers.* New York: Harper & Row.

Russell, D.H. (1984). The prevalence and seriousness of incestuous abuse. *Child Abuse and Neglect,* 8, 15-22.

Sgroi, S.M. (1982). *Handbook of clinical intervention in child sexual abuse.* Lexington, MA: Lexington Books.

Shapiro, F. (1995). *Eye movement desensitization and reprocessing: Basic principles, protocols, and procedures.* New York: Guilford Press.

Shapiro, F. (2002). *EMDR: Promises for a paradigm shift.* New York: APA Press.

Spiegel, D. and Spiegel, H. (1978). *Trance and treatment: Clinical uses of hypnosis.* Washington, DC: American Psychiatric Press.

Stamm, B. (1995). *Secondary traumatic stress: Self-care issues for clinicians, researchers, and educators.* Lutherville, MD: Sidran Press.

Steele, B.F. and Pollack, C.B. (1968). *A psychiatric study of parents who abuse infants.* Chicago: The University of Chicago Press.

Steele, K. (1989). Sitting with the shattered soul. *Journal of Psychotherapy and Personal Exploration,* 15, 19-25.

Stiver, I.P. (1991). Beyond the oedipus complex: Mothers and daughters. *Women's Growth in Connection.* Work in Progress. Wellesley, MA: Stone Center Working Paper Series.

Surrey, J.L. (1985). A theory of women's development. Work in progress. Wellesley, MA: Stone Center Working Series.

Terr, L. (1994). *Unchained memories: True stories of traumatic memories, lost and found.* New York: Basic Books.

Tower, C. (1988). *Secret scars.* New York: Penguin Books.

Ullman, S.E. (1997). Attributions, world assumptions, and recovery from sexual assault. *Journal of Child Sexual Abuse,* 6(1), 1-17.

Van der Kolk, B.A. (1996). Trauma and memory. In B.A. Van der Kolk, A.C. McFarlane, and L. Weisaeth (Eds.), *Traumatic stress* (pp. 182-213). New York: Guildford Press.

Van der Kolk, B.A. (2002). Beyond the talking cure: Somatic experience, subcortical imprints, and the treatment of trauma. In F. Shapiro, *EMDR, Promises for a paradigm shift.* New York: APA Press.

Van der Kolk, B.A. and Greenberg, M.S. (1987). The psychobiology of the trauma response: In B.A. Van der Kolk (Ed.), *Psychological trauma* (pp. 187-190). Washington, DC: American Psychiatric Press.

van Wormer, K. (2001). *Counseling female offenders and victims: A strengths-restorative approach.* New York: Springer.

Waites, E. (1993). *Trauma and survival: Post-traumatic and dissociative disorders in women.* New York: W.W. Norton and Company.

Warme, G. (1996). *The psychotherapist.* Northvale, NJ: Jason Aronson.

Wilson, J. and Lindy, J. (1994). *Countertransference in the treatment of PTSD.* New York: Guilford Press.

Wilson, J. and Raphael, B. (1993). *International handbook of traumatic stress syndromes.* New York: Plenum Press.

Winnicott, D.W. (1965). *The maturational processes and the facilitation environment: Studies in the theory of emotional development.* New York: International Universities Press.

Yeoman, B. (1999). Bad girls. *Psychology Today,* 71, 54-57.

# Index

Abandonment
    mother's fear of, 88
    survivor's feelings of, 114. *See also*
        Betrayal
Abuse
    statistics, 3
    stories
        Alana, 94-95
        Alice, 93
        Ashley, 94
        Moe, 136-137
Acceptance, survivor, 34-35
Actress, survivor as, 38-39
Acute shame. *See* Shame, survivor
ADHD, 178
Adolescence, and the mother-daughter
    relationship, 14
Adoration, of mother, 110-111, 113
Adult victims of mother-daughter
    incest, 123-132
    stories
        Alana, 124, 127, 128, 129, 130,
          131
        Ashley, 130, 132
        Iris, 128
        Lisa, 123
        Page, 126
Alcohol abuse, 66, 75-76, 104
Anger. *See also* Rage, outbursts of
    as attachment strategy, 147
    from betrayal, 96
    management of, 178
    mothers and, 86
    at societal denial of mother-daughter
        incest, 48
    when remembering abuse, 77
"Anger in connection," 165

Anxiety
    as attachment strategy, 147
    management of, 178
    as result of abuse, 78-79
Anxious avoidant attachment, 20
Anxious resistant attachment, 20
Assertiveness training, 178
Attachment behavior, 18-22
    anger as, 147
Attachment resistant, 23
Attachment theory, 18
    and the client-therapist relationship,
        22-24
Attachments, building, 147, 148,
        149-150
    ambivalence about, 160
    disruptions in, 171
Attention-deficit hyperactivity disorder
    (ADHD), 178
Avoidance, 104

Behavioral self-blame, 31
Betrayal, 27, 181
    stories
        Alana, 48-49, 50
        Beatrice, 45
        Christine, 50
        Iris, 54
        Mable, 46-47
        Sonia, 47-48, 51
Body
    acceptance of, 67
    dislike of, 33-34
Boundaries
    lack of, 111
    stories
        Jacqueline, 93

Boundaries, stories *(continued)*
    Mable, 97
    Sonia, 56, 98-99
    unlearned, 56
    violations of, 93-99, 158
Bowlby, J., 18, 20
Browne, A., 3, 27
Burning of genitals, 94
Burnout, therapist, 166
    preventing, 167
"Bystander's guilt," 163

Cast-off child, 21
Celibacy, 64-65
Chaos, invented, 96
Characterological self-blame, 31
Chodorow, N., 15
Client-therapist relationship
    and attachment theory, 22-24
Clonidine, 178
"Cognitive stage" of healing process,
    178
Cognitive-behavioral interventions, 176
Cognitive-behavioral therapy, 178
Compassion fatigue, 158
Concealment of abuse, 38. *See also*
    Secrecy
Confrontation
    survivor and abuser, 129-131
    therapist and client, 158-159
Confusion, survivor's, 39
Connectedness, lack of, 49
Control, perpetrator over victim, 38
Coperpetrator, mother as, 87-88
Coping
    difficulty with, 71-81
    stories
      Alana, 78
      Ashley, 76
      Iris, 72, 73
      Jacqueline, 75
      Lisa, 76
      Mable, 77
      Michelle, 80

Coping, stories *(continued)*
    Penny, 71
    Sonia, 79
Coping mechanisms, 42, 182
Countermanipulation, 165
Countertransference, 155-169
Crises, invented, 96

Dalenberg, C.
    on "bystander's guilt," 163
    on countertransference, 155
    on courage of therapist and client,
      169
    on PTSD in therapist's, 166
Daughters. *See* Survivor,
      mother-daughter incest
Davies, J.M., 157
Daydreaming, 74
Defensive, survivor as, 146
Denial of mother-daughter incest,
    societal, 5-6, 48, 51
Dependence on perpetrator, 110
Depression, 31, 47, 78-79
Desensitization, systematic, 178
Developmental theory, 12-15
Differentiation, 16, 55-61
Diffuse boundaries, 98
Digital penetration, 94
Disclosure
    countertransference, 164
    reluctance to, 33
Disconnection, 17
Disown mother, survivor reluctance to,
    60
Dissociation, 74, 174
Doubt. *See also* Denial of
    mother-daughter incest,
    societal
    effect of abuse, 32
    survivor's fear of, 38
Drug abuse, 75-76

Eating disorders, 74-75
EMDR, 175-177

Emotionality, 79-80
    therapist's, 155-169
Empathy, 61
Empowerment, 41-42, 52
Enema, 94
Epstein, R., 164
Erikson, E.H., 171
Exercise, 74
Exploitation, 94
Eye movement desensitization and
    reprocessing (EMDR),
    175-177

Female child, birth of, 74
Female pedophilia, literature, 5
Female therapist
    and countertransference, 141-142
    familiarity with mother-daughter
        dyad, 139-140
    guilt over healthy relationship with
        own mother, 165
    overidentifying with client, 156
    and transference, 151
Females, sex offenses by, 3-4
Femininity
    mother's, 87
    survivor's denial of, 58
Fight-or-flight, 175
Finkelhor, D., 3, 27
Fondling, 94
Fragmentation, 116
Frawley, M.G., 157

Gender, therapist's, 139-143
    stories
        Alana, 143
        Mable, 141-142
        Sonia, 142
Genesis Female Sexual Offenders
    Treatment Program, 88
Genitals, abuse of, 94
Gilbert, L., 5
Gilligan, C., 16

"Good parent" versus "bad parent,"
    therapist as, 146
Grief, 45-54
    stories
        Alana, 48-49, 50
        Beatrice, 45
        Christine, 50
        Iris, 54
        Mable, 46-47
        Sonia, 47-48, 51
Group therapy, 43, 97-98, 105-106, 178
Guided imagery, 176

Helpless, enraged victim, 157
Helplessness, therapist, 168
Herman, J.
    and dissociative state, survivor's, 74
    and group therapy, 105, 107
    and projective identification, 146
    and self-blame, 29
    and therapist's own psychological
        health, 166
    and therapy, benefits of, 183
    and transference, 162
High achiever, survivor as, 39
Hypervigilant, survivor, 149

Idealized rescuer, 157
Identification with mother, 55-61
    stories
        Ashley, 57
        Beth, 60
        Iris, 58-61
        Jacqueline, 60
        Louise, 59
        Michelle, 55-56, 59
        Patti, 58
        Taylore, 57
Identity development, impaired,
    109-117
    stories
        Alana, 109, 114
        Mable, 113
        Michelle, 111

Identity formation, 171
Individuation, 13-15, 111
Infancy, and need for relatedness, 19
Insecure attachment, 20
Insomnia, 178
Integrated treatment model, 177-179
Intimacy, fear of, 48
Invalidation of therapist, attempt at,
      151
Isolation, 37-54, 115
      stories
            Alana, 38
            Ashley, 39
            Iris, 37
            Mable, 37
            Michelle, 41
            Sonia, 41


Jordan, J.V., 16


Kaplan, A.G., 16, 139
Kegan, R., 171
Kissing, 94


Lanese, J., 135, 136
Learning disability, 110
Lesbian, survivor as, 65
Letter, survivor to self, 33
Love, abuse as act of, 88-89
Loving mother, 12
Loyalty, guilt over feelings of, 55,
      125-126


Male therapist, 141
Massage, 178
Masturbation, 66
Maternal sexual abuse. *See*
            Mother-daughter incest
Matsakis, A., 178, 179
Matthews, J., 88

Medication, therapy and, 178
Mentally ill, survivor's fear of being,
      57
Miller, A., 16
Molding, 148-149
Mother
      as abuser, 93-99. *See also*
            Mother-daughter incest
      adoration of, 110-111, 113
      childlike, 90
      confronting, 129-131
      as coperpetrator of abuse, 87-88
      emotionally needy, 85-92
      fear of abandonment, 88
      femininity of, 87
      identification with
            stories
                  Ashley, 57
                  Beth, 60
                  Iris, 58-61
                  Jacqueline, 60
                  Louise, 59
                  Michelle, 55-56, 59
                  Patti, 58
                  Taylore, 57
      love, abuse as act of, 88-89
      loyalty to, guilt over feelings of, 55,
            125-126
      parasitic, 89
      role reversal, 90, 91-92, 126-127
      step versus biological, 135-137
      stories of
            Alana, 86, 91-92
            Arabella, 90
            Ashley, 85-86
            Iris, 86
            Jan, 90-91
            Michelle, 87
            Sonia, 86-87, 88-89
            Sue, 85
      sympathy for, 86
      volatile, 86
Mother-daughter incest
      adult victims of, 123-132
      by biological mother, 135-137
      secrecy and, 94, 96, 126

Mother-daughter incest *(continued)*
  societal denial of, 5-6, 48, 51
  statistics, 3-4
  by stepmother, 135-137
  survivors. *See* Survivor,
    mother-daughter incest
  underestimation of, 4
Mother-daughter relationship
  and attachment behaviors, 18-22
  and attachment theory, 18
    and the client-therapist
      relationship, 22-24
  and developmental theory, 12-15
  differentiation from mother, 55-61
  as essential human connection,
    11-12
  identification with mother, 55-61
  and object-relations theory, 15
  and relational theory, 16-18
  repairing, 129
Motherhood
  avoiding, 59
  cultural images of, 6-7
"Mothering" therapist, 140
Mother-in-law, denying access to
    children, 121
Mourning, as part of recovery, 52, 53

Narrative therapy, 171

Object-relations theory, 15
Oral sex, 94

Parenting, survivor and, 119-121
  avoiding motherhood, 59
  denying mother-in-law access to
    children, 121
  fear of victimizing own children, 58,
    120
  female child, birth of, 74
  stories
    Alice, 119
    Ashley, 120-121

Parenting, survivor and, stories
    *(continued)*
    Mable, 120
    Michelle, 119
    Sonia, 120
Penetration with implements, 94
Perfectionist, survivor as, 39
Personality development, 171
Pharmacotherapy, 177-178
Positive thinking, 33
Post-traumatic stress disorder (PTSD),
    166, 172, 173-177
Powerlessness, survivor's feelings of,
    27, 38
Practicing phase, 13
Projection, 146, 147
Projective identification, 168
Promiscuity, 64, 66, 67
Provocative behavior, survivor to
    therapist, 152, 158
Psychological trauma, 109
"Psychologically indigestible," 136
PTSD, 166, 172, 173-177
Public complaint, making a, 43

Rage, outbursts of, 77. *See also* Anger
    split-off rage response, 149
    therapist's, 156
Reapproachment phase, 13-14
Recovery, process of, 182
Reenactment, 160-161
Relational theory, 16-18
Relationships, difficulties with, 78
Relaxation techniques, 178
Repetition compulsion, 158
Repression of feelings, survivor, 73-74,
    146
Reprocessing, 176
Rescuer, therapist as, 161-162
Role reversal, 90, 91-92, 126-127
Rosencrans, B., 7

Sadistic abuser, 157
Scrubbing of genitals, 94

Second adolescence, 115
Secrecy, 94, 96, 126. *See also* Shame,
     survivor
Seducer and the seduced, 157
Selective serotonin reuptake inhibitors
     (SSRIs), 178
Self-blame, 29-31, 50, 57
     stories, Soulitsa and Val, 31
Self-criticism, 33
Self-definition, 14
Self-destructive behavior, 71, 72, 104
Self-injurious behavior, 32, 158
Self-in-relation theory, 16-18
Self-model, child's, 19
Self-mutilation, 76
Self-talk, 178
Separation, process of, 13-15, 111
Separation anxiety, 58
Sex play, 66
Sexual countertransference, 163
Sexual orientation, confusion about, 64,
     65
Sexuality, impaired
     stories
          Ashley, 65
          Christine, 66
          Iris, 63, 65
          Lisa, 63
          Mable, 65, 67
          Michelle, 69
          Taylore, 66
Shame, survivor
     acute, 27-35, 68
     secrecy and, 8, 104. *See also*
          Secrecy
     stories
          Christine, 34
          Jan, 27
          Mable, 28-29
          Michelle, 103
          Patti, 103
          Sonia, 32
     therapy as source of, 162
"Shame trap," 125
Silence, survivor, 7-8, 40, 182-183. *See
     also* Secrecy; Shame, survivor

Societal denial of mother-daughter
     incest, 5-6, 48, 51
Sovereign nation, family as, 5
Speechless, survivor as, 52
Spiegel, D., 158
Spiegel, H., 158
Split-off rage response, 149
Stepmother, as abuser, 135-137
Stigmatization, 7-8, 27, 112
     stories
          Ashley, 105
          Elsie, 106
          Michelle, 103
          Patti, 103, 104
          Sonia, 106
Stiver, I.P., 16
Stress inoculation training, 178
"Stuck" in therapy, 165
Suicide, 52, 104, 158
     story, Alana, 39-40
Support group, therapist, 167
Support system, for therapist, 167
Surrey, J.L., 16
Survivor, mother-daughter incest
     and alcohol abuse, 66
     and betrayal, feelings of, 45-54
     confronting abuser, 129-131
     coping, difficulty with, 71-81
     differentiation from mother, 55-61
     fear of victimizing own children, 58,
          120
     and friends, prevented from making,
          90-91
     and grief, 45-54
     identification with mother, 55-61
     and isolation, 37-54
     and parenting, 119-121
     and promiscuity, 64, 66, 67
     and role reversal, 90, 91-92,
          126-127
     and sexuality, impaired, 63-69
     and shame, 8, 27-35, 68
     silence, 7-8, 40, 182-183
     stigmatization, 7-8
     stories. *See* Survivor stories
     sympathy for mother, 86

Survivor, mother-daughter incest
  *(continued)*
  trust, regaining, 48, 68, 95-96
  victimization, potential for further,
    66, 78
Survivor stories
  Alana
    adult victim, 124, 127, 128, 129,
      130, 131
    and betrayal/grief, 48-49, 50
    and coping, 78
    describes abuse, 94-95
    describes mother, 86, 91-92
    and gender of therapist, 143
    and identity development, 109,
      114
    and isolation, 38
    suicide attempt, 39-40
  Alice
    describes abuse, 93
    and parenting, 119
  Arabella, describes mother, 90
  Ashley
    adult victim, 130, 132
    and coping, 76
    describes abuse, 94
    describes mother, 85-86
    identification with mother, 57
    and isolation, 39
    and parenting, 120-121
    and sexuality, 65
    and stigmatization, 105
  Beatrice, and betrayal/grief, 45
  Beth, and identification with
      mother, 60
  Christine
    and betrayal/grief, 50
    and sexuality, 66
    on shame, 34
  Elsie, and stigmatization, 106
  Gloria, and betrayal/grief, 54
  Iris
    adult victim, 128
    and betrayal/grief, 54
    and coping, 72, 73
    describes mother, 86

Survivor stories, Iris *(continued)*
    identification with mother, 58, 61
    and isolation, 37
    and sexuality, 63, 65
  Jacqueline
    and boundary violations, 93
    and coping, 75
    identification with mother, 60
  Jan
    describes mother, 90-91
    on shame, 27
  Lisa
    adult victim, 123
    and coping, 76
    and sexuality, 63
  Louise
    identification with mother, 59
    and isolation, 40
  Mable
    and betrayal/grief, 46-47
    and boundaries, 97
    and coping, 77
    and gender of therapist, 141-142
    and identity development, 113
    and isolation, 37
    and parenting, 120
    and sexuality, 65, 67
    on shame, 28-29
  Michelle
    and coping, 80
    describes mother, 87
    and identification with mother,
      55-56, 59
    and identity development, 111
    and isolation, 41
    and parenting, 119
    and sexuality, 69
    and stigmatization, 103
  Moe, describes feelings about abuse,
    136-137
  Page, adult victim, 126
  Patti
    identification with mother, 58
    and stigmatization, 103, 104
  Penny, and coping, 71

Survivor stories, Sonia *(continued)*
    and betrayal/grief, 47-48, 51
    and boundaries, 56, 98-99
    and coping, 79
    describes mother, 86-87, 88-89
    and gender of therapist, 142
    and isolation, 41
    and parenting, 120
    on self-blame, 30-31
    on shame, 32
    and stigmatization, 106
   Soulitsa, on self-blame, 31
   Sue, describes mother, 85
   Taylore
    identification with mother, 57
    on mother-child bond, 135
    and sexuality, 66
   Val, on self-blame, 31
Symbiosis, 13
Sympathy, for mother, 86

"Target experience," 176
Termination, therapy, 149
Therapist
   accused of being a seducer, 150
   acting out negative feelings toward,
    150
   as ally, 152
   blaming the, 150
   burnout, 166
    preventing, 167
   and compassion fatigue, 158
   confronting client, 158
   and countertransference, 155-169
   emotionality, 155-169
   female
    and countertransference, 141-142
    familiarity with mother-daughter
     dyad, 139-140
    guilt over healthy relationship
     with own mother, 165
    overidentifying with client, 156
    and transference, 151
   gender, 139-143

Therapist, gender *(continued)*
   stories
    Alana, 143
    Mable, 141-142
    Sonia, 142
   as "good parent" versus "bad
    parent," 146
   helplessness, 168
   invalidation of, attempt at, 151
   male, 141
   openness to mother-daughter incest,
    44
   and PTSD, 166
   rage and, 156
   as rescuer, 161-162
   sexual advances to, 152, 158
   support groups for, 167
   support system for, 167
   threats to, 152
   transference to, 145-147
Therapy, with survivors
   adult victims, 123-132
   developmental issues, 60
   group, 43, 97-98, 105-106, 178
   and identity development, 109-117
   integrated treatment model, 177-179
   and medication, 178
   paradigms found in, 157
   and parenting, 119-121
   and post-traumatic stress disorder
    (PTSD), 172, 173-177
   repairing mother-daughter
    relationship, 129
   as source of shame, 162
   and stigmatization, 103-107
   termination of, 149
   theoretical frameworks, 171-173
   transference and, 145-153
Tower, C., 65
Transference, 145-153
"Trap of daughterhood," 5
"Trap of parenthood," 6
Traumatic countertransference, 155
Traumatic sexualization, 27
Traumatization, victim, 27

Trust, regaining, 48, 68, 95-96
"Tuning out and turning off," 77

Underestimation, mother-daughter
    incest, 4
Underpants, 94
Unseen, neglected child, 157

Vicarious traumatization, 155
Volatile, mother as, 86
Voyeurism, 94

Water, held under, 94
Webster, P., 5
Withdrawal, countertransference, 164,
    165
"Witness guilt," 165

*THE HAWORTH MALTREATMENT AND TRAUMA PRESS®*
Robert A. Geffner, PhD
Senior Editor

**MUNCHAUSEN BY PROXY: IDENTIFICATION, INTERVENTION, AND CASE MANAGEMENT** by Louisa J. Lasher and Mary S. Sheridan. (2004). "This book is an excellent resource for professionals from all disciplines who may be confronted with this misunderstood disorder. Any question one would have regarding MSP—from the initial identification to assisting victim with treatment—is thoroughly addressed. This book is a must for every professional involved in MBP investigations." *Larry C. Brubaker, FBI Special Agent (retired)*

**MOTHER-DAUGHTER INCEST: A GUIDE FOR HELPING PROFESSIONALS** by Beverly A. Ogilvie. (2004). "Beverly A. Ogilvie has succeeded in writing what will become the definitive resource for therapists working with mother-daughter incest. Ogilvie presents a solid theoretical background, blending developmental, object-relations, self-in-relation, and attachment theories to explain the dynamics of this rare but devastating abuse. The book moves beyond theory and provides a working model to guide therapists working in this area." *Gina M. Pallotta, PhD, Associate Professor of Psychology and Clinical Graduate Director, California State University, Stanislaus*

**REBUILDING ATTACHMENTS WITH TRAUMATIZED CHILDREN: HEALING FROM LOSSES, VIOLENCE, ABUSE, AND NEGLECT** by Richard Kagan. (2004). "Dr. Richard Kagan, a recognized expert in working with traumatized children, has written a truly impressive book. Not only does the book contain a wealth of information for understanding the complex issues faced by traumatized youngsters, but it also offers specific interventions that can be used to help these children and their caregivers become more hopeful and resilient. . . . I am certain that this book will be read and reread by professionals engaged in improving the lives of at-risk youth." *Robert Brooks, PhD, Faculty, Harvard Medical School and author of* Raising Resilient Children *and* The Power of Resilience

**PSYCHOLOGICAL TRAUMA AND THE DEVELOPING BRAIN: NEUROLOGICALLY BASED INTERVENTIONS FOR TROUBLED CHILDREN** by Phyllis T. Stien and Joshua C. Kendall. (2003). "Stien and Kendall provide us with a great service. In this clearly written and important book, they synthesize a wealth of crucial information that links childhood trauma to brain abnormalities and subsequent mental illness. Equally important, they show us how the trauma also affects the child's social and intellectual development. I recommend this book to all clinicians and administrators." *Charles L. Whitfield, MD, Author of* The Truth About Depression *and* The Truth About Mental Illness

**CHILD MALTREATMENT RISK ASSESSMENTS: AN EVALUATION GUIDE** by Sue Righthand, Bruce Kerr, and Kerry Drach. (2003). "This book is essential reading for clinicians and forensic examiners who see cases involving issues related to child maltreatment. The authors have compiled an impressive critical survey of the relevant research on child maltreatment. Their material is well organized into sections on definitions, impact, risk assessment, and risk management. This book represents a giant step toward promoting evidence-based evaluations, treatment, and testimony." *Diane H. Schetky, MD, Professor of Psychiatry, University of Vermont College of Medicine*

**SIMPLE AND COMPLEX POST-TRAUMATIC STRESS DISORDER: STRATEGIES FOR COMPREHENSIVE TREATMENT IN CLINICAL PRACTICE** edited by Mary Beth Williams and John F. Sommer Jr. (2002). "A welcome addition to the literature on treating survivors of traumatic events, this volume possesses all the ingredients necessary for even the experienced clinician to master the management of patients with PTSD." *Terence M. Keane, PhD, Chief, Psychology Service, VA Boston Healthcare System; Professor and Vice Chair of Research in Psychiatry, Boston University School of Medicine*

**FOR LOVE OF COUNTRY: CONFRONTING RAPE AND SEXUAL HARASSMENT IN THE U.S. MILITARY** by T. S. Nelson. (2002). "Nelson brings an important message—that the absence of current media attention doesn't mean the problem has gone away; that only decisive action by military leadership at all levels can break the cycle of repeated traumatization; and that the failure to do so is, as Nelson puts it, a 'power failure'—a refusal to exert positive leadership at all levels to stop violent individuals from using the worst power imaginable." *Chris Lombardi, Correspondent, Women's E-News, New York City*

**THE INSIDERS: A MAN'S RECOVERY FROM TRAUMATIC CHILDHOOD ABUSE** by Robert Blackburn Knight. (2002). "An important book. . . . Fills a gap in the literature about healing from childhood sexual abuse by allowing us to hear, in undiluted terms, about one man's history and journey of recovery." *Amy Pine, MA, LMFT, psychotherapist and co-founder, Survivors Healing Center, Santa Cruz, California*

**WE ARE NOT ALONE: A GUIDEBOOK FOR HELPING PROFESSIONALS AND PARENTS SUPPORTING ADOLESCENT VICTIMS OF SEXUAL ABUSE** by Jade Christine Angelica. (2002). "Encourages victims and their families to participate in the system in an effort to heal from their victimization, seek justice, and hold offenders accountable for their crimes. An exceedingly vital training tool." *Janet Fine, MS, Director, Victim Witness Assistance Program and Children's Advocacy Center, Suffolk County District Attorney's Office, Boston*

**WE ARE NOT ALONE: A TEENAGE GIRL'S PERSONAL ACCOUNT OF INCEST FROM DISCLOSURE THROUGH PROSECUTION AND TREATMENT** by Jade Christine Angelica. (2002). "A valuable resource for teens who have been sexually abused and their parents. With compassion and eloquent prose, Angelica walks people through the criminal justice system—from disclosure to final outcome." *Kathleen Kendall-Tackett, PhD, Research Associate, Family Research Laboratory, University of New Hampshire, Durham*

**WE ARE NOT ALONE: A TEENAGE BOY'S PERSONAL ACCOUNT OF CHILD SEXUAL ABUSE FROM DISCLOSURE THROUGH PROSECUTION AND TREATMENT** by Jade Christine Angelica. (2002). "Inspires us to work harder to meet kids' needs, answer their questions, calm their fears, and protect them from their abusers and the system, which is often not designed to respond to them in a language they understand." *Kevin L. Ryle, JD, Assistant District Attorney, Middlesex, Massachusetts*

**GROWING FREE: A MANUAL FOR SURVIVORS OF DOMESTIC VIOLENCE** by Wendy Susan Deaton and Michael Hertica. (2001). "This is a necessary book for anyone who is scared and starting to think about what it would take to 'grow free.' . . . Very helpful for friends and relatives of a person in a domestic violence situation. I recommend it highly." *Colleen Friend, LCSW, Field Work Consultant, UCLA Department of Social Welfare, School of Public Policy & Social Research*

**A THERAPIST'S GUIDE TO GROWING FREE: A MANUAL FOR SURVIVORS OF DOMESTIC VIOLENCE** by Wendy Susan Deaton and Michael Hertica. (2001). "An excellent synopsis of the theories and research behind the manual." *Beatrice Crofts Yorker, RN, JD, Professor of Nursing, Georgia State University, Decatur*

**PATTERNS OF CHILD ABUSE: HOW DYSFUNCTIONAL TRANSACTIONS ARE REPLICATED IN INDIVIDUALS, FAMILIES, AND THE CHILD WELFARE SYSTEM** by Michael Karson. (2001). "No one interested in what may well be the major public health epidemic of our time in terms of its long-term consequences for our society can afford to pass up the opportunity to read this enlightening work." *Howard Wolowitz, PhD, Professor Emeritus, Psychology Department, University of Michigan, Ann Arbor*

**IDENTIFYING CHILD MOLESTERS: PREVENTING CHILD SEXUAL ABUSE BY RECOGNIZING THE PATTERNS OF THE OFFENDERS** by Carla van Dam. (2000). "The definitive work on the subject. . . . Provides parents and others with the tools to recognize when and how to intervene." *Roger W. Wolfe, MA, Co-Director, N. W. Treatment Associates, Seattle, Washington*

**POLITICAL VIOLENCE AND THE PALESTINIAN FAMILY: IMPLICATIONS FOR MENTAL HEALTH AND WELL-BEING** by Vivian Khamis. (2000). "A valuable book . . . a pioneering work that fills a glaring gap in the study of Palestinian society." *Elia Zureik, Professor of Sociology, Queens University, Kingston, Ontario, Canada*

**STOPPING THE VIOLENCE: A GROUP MODEL TO CHANGE MEN'S ABUSIVE ATTITUDES AND BEHAVIORS** by David J. Decker. (1999). "A concise and thorough manual to assist clinicians in learning the causes and dynamics of domestic violence." *Joanne Kittel, MSW, LICSW, Yachats, Oregon*

**STOPPING THE VIOLENCE: A GROUP MODEL TO CHANGE MEN'S ABUSIVE ATTITUDES AND BEHAVIORS, THE CLIENT WORKBOOK** by David J. Decker. (1999).

**BREAKING THE SILENCE: GROUP THERAPY FOR CHILDHOOD SEXUAL ABUSE, A PRACTITIONER'S MANUAL** by Judith A. Margolin. (1999). "This book is an extremely valuable and well-written resource for all therapists working with adult survivors of child sexual abuse." *Esther Deblinger, PhD, Associate Professor of Clinical Psychiatry, University of Medicine and Dentistry of New Jersey School of Osteopathic Medicine*

**"I NEVER TOLD ANYONE THIS BEFORE": MANAGING THE INITIAL DISCLOSURE OF SEXUAL ABUSE RE-COLLECTIONS** by Janice A. Gasker. (1999). "Discusses the elements needed to create a safe, therapeutic environment and offers the practitioner a number of useful strategies for responding appropriately to client disclosure." *Roberta G. Sands, PhD, Associate Professor, University of Pennsylvania School of Social Work*

**FROM SURVIVING TO THRIVING: A THERAPIST'S GUIDE TO STAGE II RECOVERY FOR SURVIVORS OF CHILDHOOD ABUSE** by Mary Bratton. (1999). "A must read for all, including survivors. Bratton takes a lifelong debilitating disorder and unravels its intricacies in concise, succinct, and understandable language." *Phillip A. Whitner, PhD, Sr. Staff Counselor, University Counseling Center, The University of Toledo, Ohio*

**SIBLING ABUSE TRAUMA: ASSESSMENT AND INTERVENTION STRATEGIES FOR CHILDREN, FAMILIES, AND ADULTS** by John V. Caffaro and Allison Conn-Caffaro. (1998). "One area that has almost consistently been ignored in the research and writing on child maltreatment is the area of sibling abuse. This book is a welcome and required addition to the developing literature on abuse." *Judith L. Alpert, PhD, Professor of Applied Psychology, New York University*

**BEARING WITNESS: VIOLENCE AND COLLECTIVE RESPONSIBILITY** by Sandra L. Bloom and Michael Reichert. (1998). "A totally convincing argument. . . . Demands careful study by all elected representatives, the clergy, the mental health and medical professions, representatives of the media, and all those unwittingly involved in this repressive perpetuation and catastrophic global problem." *Harold I. Eist, MD, Past President, American Psychiatric Association*

**TREATING CHILDREN WITH SEXUALLY ABUSIVE BEHAVIOR PROBLEMS: GUIDELINES FOR CHILD AND PARENT INTERVENTION** by Jan Ellen Burton, Lucinda A. Rasmussen, Julie Bradshaw, Barbara J. Christopherson, and Steven C. Huke. (1998). "An extremely readable book that is well-documented and a mine of valuable 'hands on' information. . . . This is a book that all those who work with sexually abusive children or want to work with them must read." *Sharon K. Araji, PhD, Professor of Sociology, University of Alaska, Anchorage*

**THE LEARNING ABOUT MYSELF (LAMS) PROGRAM FOR AT-RISK PARENTS: LEARNING FROM THE PAST—CHANGING THE FUTURE** by Verna Rickard. (1998). "This program should be a part of the resource materials of every mental health professional trusted with the responsibility of working with 'at-risk' parents." *Terry King, PhD, Clinical Psychologist, Federal Bureau of Prisons, Catlettsburg, Kentucky*

**THE LEARNING ABOUT MYSELF (LAMS) PROGRAM FOR AT-RISK PARENTS: HANDBOOK FOR GROUP PARTICIPANTS** by Verna Rickard. (1998). "Not only is the LAMS program designed to be educational and build skills for future use, it is also fun!" *Martha Morrison Dore, PhD, Associate Professor of Social Work, Columbia University, New York*

**BRIDGING WORLDS: UNDERSTANDING AND FACILITATING ADOLESCENT RECOVERY FROM THE TRAUMA OF ABUSE** by Joycee Kennedy and Carol McCarthy. (1998). "An extraordinary survey of the history of child neglect and abuse in America. . . . A wonderful teaching tool at the university level, but should be required reading in high schools as well." *Florabel Kinsler, PhD, BCD, LCSW, Licensed Clinical Social Worker, Los Angeles, California*

**CEDAR HOUSE: A MODEL CHILD ABUSE TREATMENT PROGRAM** by Bobbi Kendig with Clara Lowry. (1998). "Kendig and Lowry truly . . . realize the saying that we are our brothers' keepers. Their spirit permeates this volume, and that spirit of caring is what always makes the difference for people in painful situations." *Hershel K. Swinger, PhD, Clinical Director, Children's Institute International, Los Angeles, California*

**SEXUAL, PHYSICAL, AND EMOTIONAL ABUSE IN OUT-OF-HOME CARE: PREVENTION SKILLS FOR AT-RISK CHILDREN** by Toni Cavanagh Johnson and Associates. (1997). "Professionals who make dispositional decisions or who are related to out-of-home care for children could benefit from reading and following the curriculum of this book with children in placements." *Issues in Child Abuse Accusations*